Pharmacy Master
The Ultimate BCGP Review

Author
Eric Christianson, Pharm.D., BCPS, BCGP

Looking for more BCGP Study Material? Get an exclusive 35% off the CGP Practice exam AND 10+ hour online webinar series!

Go to
https://www.meded101.com/pharmacist-board-certification-study-material/

Use discount code bcgpbook at checkout!

Copyright and Disclaimer

Copyright © Eric Christianson 2016

All rights reserved. It is not permitted to reproduce, distribute, or transmit in any form or by any means the content in this book without the written permission of the publisher except in the case of brief quotations as allowed by copyright law.

This book is for educational purposes only. It is not intended to diagnose, treat or be construed as medical advice in anyway. This book is not intended as a substitute for sound medical advice from a pharmacist, physician, nurse, or other qualified healthcare professional. Please consult the appropriate healthcare professional in matters relating to your health and any symptom that may require diagnosis, treatment, or medical attention.

The author has made every effort to make sure the information in this book is correct at time of release. However, the author and publisher do not assume and hereby disclaim any liability to any party for loss, damage, or disruption caused by any errors or omissions in this book. Whether the errors or omissions were a result of negligence, accident, or any other cause, the author does not assume and hereby disclaims liability.

The Board Certified Geriatric Pharmacist is a designation from the Board of Pharmacy Specialties and formerly a designation from the Commission for Certification in Geriatric Pharmacy. The designation from the CCGP was formerly called the CGP credential. The contents within this study guide are not affiliated or endorsed by either organization.

Cover Illustration and Design Copyright 2016 by: Melissa Christianson

Formatting by: Melissa Christianson

ABOUT THE AUTHOR

Eric Christianson, Pharm.D., BCPS, BCGP is a clinical pharmacist who is passionate about medication education and patient safety. Eric is the founder of meded101.com, a website dedicated to providing quality, real world medication education for healthcare professionals. He has been acknowledged by The Wall Street Journal, American Journal of Nursing, National Association Directors of Nursing, Pharmacy Podcast, Pharmacy Today, and Pharmacy Times.

Essential Tremor	57
Failure to Thrive	58
Falls in the Elderly	59
Generalized Anxiety Disorder	61
GERD	63
Geriatric Vaccines	65
Glaucoma	67
Gout	69
Headaches	71
HIV/AIDS	73
Hyperlipidemia	75
Hypertension	77
Hyperthyroid	80
Hypokalemia	81
Hyponatremia	82
Hypothyroid	84
Influenza	86
Insomnia	88
Irritable Bowel Syndrome	90
Malnutrition	92
Menopause Complications	93
Multiple Sclerosis	95
Nausea/Vomiting	97
Neuropathy	99
Oncology Complications	101
Orthostasis	103
Osteoarthritis	105
Osteomyelitis	109
Osteoporosis	111

Contents

Acute Coronary Syndrome 8
Acute Kidney Injury (Acute Renal Failure) 10
Allergic Rhinitis 12
Anemia 13
Asthma 15
Atopic Dermatitis 18
Atrial Fibrillation 19
Bacterial/Viral Eye Infection 21
Biostatistics Basics 22
Bipolar Disorder 24
BPH 27
Cholelithiasis 28
Chronic Kidney Disease 29
Cirrhosis 31
Clostridium Difficile (C. Diff.) 33
Common Drug Resistant Bacteria 34
Congestive Heart Failure 35
Constipation 37
COPD 39
Coronary Artery Disease 41
Crohn's Disease 42
Deep Vein Thrombosis/Pulmonary Embolism 44
Delirium 47
Dementia 49
Dementia Related Behaviors 51
Depression 53
Dysphagia 55

Pancreatitis 113

Parkinson's Disorder 114

Peptic Ulcer Disease 116

Peripheral Artery Disease 118

Physiological and Lifestyle Changes in the Elderly 119

Pneumonia 122

Restless Legs 124

Rheumatoid Arthritis 126

Schizophrenia 128

Seizures 130

Sexual Dysfunction 132

Shingles 133

Skin and Soft Tissue Infection 135

Smoking Cessation 136

Stroke/TIA 137

Type 2 Diabetes 139

Ulcerative Colitis 144

Urinary Incontinence 145

Urinary Tract Infections 147

Critical Guidelines/References/Resources 150

Acute Coronary Syndrome

Signs/Symptoms/Diagnosis/Complications
- Blockage of blood flow in the coronary artery
    - Clot formation/plaque buildup
- Chest pain
- Pressure on chest
- May present with atypical symptoms in females/elderly
    - Arm pain
    - Back pain
    - Fatigue
    - CNS changes
- Light headed, dizziness
- Possible nausea and vomiting
- STEMI
    - Cardiac Biomarkers elevated
        - Troponin, CK-MB
        - Indicates cardiac damage
    - S-T segment elevation upon EKG review
    - Highest severity MI
- Non-STEMI
    - Biomarkers positive
    - S-T segment is unchanged upon EKG review
- Unstable Angina
    - Symptoms similar to MI
    - No biomarkers

Common Risk Factors
- Age
    - Men > 45, women > 55
- Tobacco
- Diabetes
- High blood pressure
- Dyslipidemia
- Family history
- Obesity/lack of physical activity
- Use of stimulants like cocaine, amphetamines

Medications to Know
- Aspirin
    - Always a drug of choice for prevention
    - Also used in acute treatment/emergency situation

- Clopidogrel
    - Used in combination with aspirin or alternative for those who can't tolerate aspirin
    - Usually for 6-12 months following stenting
        - May be shorter for high risk bleeding complications
        - May be longer if multiple MI's or MI that happened while patient was on aspirin alone, based upon clinical judgement
        - Important to reassess risk/benefit of continuing clopidogrel and aspirin at 6-12 month mark and/or if encountering bleeding risk
    - Prodrug
        - 2C19 converts to active form
        - Rapid metabolizers may be at higher risk of bleed
        - Slow metabolizers may have risk of non-response or increased risk of clot formation/MI
        - Omeprazole can inhibit 2C19 – clinical impact still debated/controversial
- Statin Therapy
    - High intensity statin for most unless intolerant
- ACE Inhibitors or ARB
    - Appropriate post MI as tolerated
- Beta-blockers
    - Appropriate post MI as tolerated

Acute Kidney Injury (Acute Renal Failure)

Signs/Symptoms/Diagnosis/Complications
- Usually change in urine output
- Rise in creatinine is typical
- Rise in blood urea nitrogen (BUN)
- Fluid accumulation (edema)
- CNS changes
- Possible electrolyte imbalances
- Risk that AKI can cause permanent renal failure
- Numerous possible causes
    - Dehydration
    - Obstruction
    - Drugs
    - Infection
    - Bladder/kidney cancer
    - Lupus

Common Risk Factors
- Underlying chronic kidney disease
- Age
- Diabetes
- Hypertension
- Drugs

Medications to Know
- No medications to "treat" acute renal failure
- Dialysis is used to filter blood where normal function can't expeditiously be restored
- Treat underlying cause if possible
    - I.e. infection -> antibiotics, dehydration -> fluid replacement etc.
- Correct imbalances caused by acute renal failure
    - I.e. hyperkalemia
        - Sodium Polystyrene Sulfonate
            - GI side effects
    - In emergency setting may see insulin utilized to bring down K+
- Drugs known to cause/contribute to AKI
    - Vancomycin
    - Aminoglycosides
    - NSAIDs

- ACE/ARBS
- Contrast dye
- Amphotericin B
- Chemo agents (i.e. Platinum compounds)
- Diuretics via dehydration risk

Allergic Rhinitis

Signs/Symptoms/Diagnosis/Complications
- Runny nose
- Sneezing
- Red, itchy eyes
- Sinus pressure
- Coughing
- Sore throat

Common Risk Factors
- Family history
- Exposure to allergens

Medications to Know
- Nasal corticosteroids (i.e. fluticasone)
    - Usual first line
    - Side effects (overall usually well tolerated)
        - Taste disturbance, nasal irritation
- Antihistamines
    - 2nd generation (loratadine, cetirizine etc.)
        - Sedation, dry mouth SE's
        - Usually much better tolerated than 1st generation
    - 1st generation (diphenhydramine, doxylamine, etc.)
        - Highly anticholinergic
        - Not first line, especially in the elderly
        - If itching or skin reactions, you may see 1st generation medications used more often
    - Oral Decongestants (pseudoephedrine and phenylephrine)
        - Can raise blood pressure
        - Contribute to urinary retention (i.e. patients with BPH)
        - Possibly increase anxiety/insomnia
        - Minimize use if possible in the elderly (short duration if necessary)
    - Nasal Decongestant
        - Oxymetazoline
        - Use only for 3 days max
        - Risk of rebound congestion
    - Nasal saline
        - Minimal to no side effects
        - Can help with symptoms, irritation

Anemia

Signs/Symptoms/Diagnosis/Complications
- Fatigue
- Weakness
- Orthostasis
- Dizziness
- Pale skin
- Poor blood flow/cold extremities
- Types of anemia (lack, shortage, or loss of red blood cell production)
    - Pernicious
        - Caused by B12 deficiency, lack of absorption
        - High mean corpuscular volume (MCV) may be indicative often termed megaloblastic
    - Folic acid deficiency
        - Also megaloblastic
    - Iron deficiency
        - Absorption or diet causes most common
        - Low MCV may be indicative
        - Ferritin monitored in the elderly
    - Blood loss
        - GI bleed, trauma, etc.
    - Kidney disease
        - Damage to the kidney which produces erythropoietin
        - Erythropoietin stimulates the production of red blood cells
        - Patients will often have an elevated creatinine
    - Rare bone marrow disorders

Common Risk Factors
- Diet changes/malnutrition
- CKD
- Chemotherapy
- Family history
- Age

Medications to Know
- Vitamin B-12
    - Treatment of pernicious
    - Oral absorption may be limited due to loss of intrinsic factor in elderly patients
    - Often may supplement with injectable B12 – "B12 shots"

- - Blood levels of homocysteine and methylmalonic acid in addition to B12 may be monitored
  - Supplementation well tolerated
  - Minimal to no risk of over supplementation
- Folic acid deficiency can also contribute to megaloblastic anemia
  - Replacement may be necessary if deficiency
  - Well tolerated, minimal to no risk of over supplementation
- Iron supplements
  - Ferrous fumarate has highest elemental > sulfate > gluconate
  - Constipation
  - Black stools
  - Binding interactions (i.e. levothyroxine, quinolones, tetracyclines)
  - Vitamin C may aid absorption
  - Polysaccharide iron complex may be an option if not enough absorption from standard therapy
  - Remember to assess iron if erythropoietin stimulating agents are used
- ESA's (erythropoietin stimulating agents)
  - Boxed warning for cardiovascular events
  - Can exacerbate hypertension
  - Injection only
  - Lack of iron stores is common reason for response in hemoglobin
  - Use primarily in oncology or possibly CKD due to lack of endogenous erythropoietin
- PPI's (see GERD for further details)
  - Will often be used for prophylaxis, prevention of GI bleed/anemia
    - NSAIDs
    - Steroids (oral)
- Transfusion – way to quickly raise hemoglobin

Asthma

Signs/Symptoms/Diagnosis/Complications
- Reactive airway disease
- Wheezing
- Coughing, nighttime awakenings
- Assess frequency of exacerbations
    - Use of prn short acting (i.e. albuterol)
    - Nighttime awakenings
    - ER or hospitalizations
- Often caused by triggers
    - Exercise
    - Cold air
    - Infection
    - Environmental allergies
    - GERD
    - Medications (i.e. beta-blockers)
- Spirometry, Peak flow, and methacholine testing may be done to assess diagnosis and/or disease severity (usually diagnosed at younger ages)
- Intermittent Asthma – General Rule of Two
    - Symptoms 2 or less days per week
    - Nighttime awakenings 2 or less days per month
    - Use of short acting beta agonist (SABA) 2 or less times per week – do not include anticipated use for exercise induced asthma
    - No limit on physical activity
- Mild Persistent
    - Symptoms 3+x's per week, but not daily
    - 3-4 nighttime awakenings per month
- Moderate Persistent
    - Daily symptoms
    - More than 1x/week (nighttime symptoms)
    - FEV1 60-80% of predicted
- Severe Persistent
    - Symptoms all throughout the day
    - Often daily nighttime awakenings
    - Severe limitation on physical activity
    - FEV1 <60% of predicted
- Rapid reversal with short acting beta-agonists (albuterol)

Common Risk Factors
- Exposure to second hand smoke

- Allergies
- Obese
- Exposure to airborne chemical
- Smoking
- Family history

Medications to Know
- Medication workflow with increasing severity of asthma
    - SABA->add Inhaled corticosteroid->add LABA, increase inhaled corticosteroid dose or add leukotriene modifiers (i.e. montelukast)->theophylline, systemic corticosteroids
    - Systemic corticosteroids for acute exacerbations
    - Inhaled anticholinergics may be tried if struggling to find a regimen that is working, but most often only used for COPD
- SABA (short acting beta agonists)
    - Albuterol, Levalbuterol
    - Acute relief of respiratory distress
    - AE's – shakiness, tremor, tachycardia
    - Potential impact of reducing serum potassium, but rarely clinically significant with inhaled medications
    - Monitoring use of SABA in asthma is very important to assessing severity/staging of asthma
- Inhaled corticosteroids
    - Budesonide, fluticasone
    - Take time to work (not meant for acute relief)
    - Reduce inflammation
    - Increased risk of thrush (rinsing important)
    - Long term concerns are not as big of a deal with inhaled corticosteroids compared to systemic corticosteroids
- LABA (long acting beta agonists)
    - Formoterol
    - Never use alone in asthma
    - Often added on to inhaled corticosteroid for patients who need more control
    - Similar adverse effect profile to short acting beta agonists (same mechanism, just longer duration of action)
    - Do not use for acute relief
- Leukotriene modifiers
    - Montelukast
    - Oral option
    - Can be helpful for allergies as well

- - Post marketing case reports of psych/behavioral related changes
- Theophylline
  - Last line therapy
  - Monitoring of drug levels (target usually 5-15)
  - Lots of drug interactions through CYP1A2
  - Lots of systemic effects
    - Similar effects to caffeine, GI, tachycardia, tremor, insomnia, anxiety

Atopic Dermatitis

Signs/Symptoms/Diagnosis/Complications
- Itching
- Redness
- Swelling
- Usually in the creases of the body (behind the knee, inside the elbow area)
- Risk of open sores from itching, bleeding, infection

Common Risk Factors
- History of allergies

Medications/Treatments to Know
- Avoid irritants
- Corticosteroid creams
    - A few potency examples - in order of least potent to most
    - Hydrocortisone 1%
    - Triamcinolone 0.25%
    - Clobetasol propionate 0.05%
- Calcineurin inhibitors
    - Tacrolimus
- For severe cases, may see systemic therapy given short term
    - Corticosteroids
    - Antihistamines

Atrial Fibrillation

Signs/Symptoms/Diagnosis/Complications
- Classifications
    - Paroxysmal (occasional), spontaneously resolves itself
    - Persistent
    - Permanent
- Fluttering in the chest
- Feeling faint, weakness, syncope
- Risk of thromboembolic stroke
- EKG used to assess diagnosis

Common Risk Factors
- Chads2Vasc – Score of 2 or greater indications that anticoagulation should be used to prevent stroke due to atrial fibrillation
    - CHF +1
    - Hypertension +1
    - Age >65 +1, >75 +2
    - Diabetes +1
    - Sex: Female +1
    - Vascular disease +1
    - Stroke/TIA +2

Medications to Know
- Rate control is primary goal
    - Cardioselective beta blocker is often initial choice (especially if compelling indications like CHF or angina) i.e. metoprolol
        - See hypertension for more details on beta-blockers
    - Calcium channel blocker (non-dihydropyridine) – work to slow the heart rate in atrial fibrillation i.e. diltiazem, verapamil
        - Caution in CHF, can exacerbate edema/fluid retention
        - See hypertension for more details on calcium channel blockers
    - Digoxin
        - May see a loading dose used for atrial fibrillation (typically not in CHF)
        - Might be a possible choice in a patient who has low blood pressure and may not be able to tolerate B-Blocker or CCB
        - Target goal concentration generally higher for atrial fibrillation versus CHF
            - Around 0.8-1.2 (versus 0.5 to 0.8 for CHF)

- Signs of toxicity – weight loss, poor appetite, GI upset, low pulse, central nervous system changes
- Can accumulate with worsening kidney function
- Can cause arrhythmias; low potassium or low magnesium levels can potentially increase this risk
- Amiodarone can increase digoxin levels
- Antiarrhythmics
    - Amiodarone
        - Controls rhythm
        - Extremely long half-life; effects can linger a long time following discontinuation
        - Also be on the lookout for drug interactions being complicated by this long half life
        - Monitor thyroid function (hypothyroid more common than hyperthyroid)
        - Can cause pulmonary fibrosis, monitor lung function throughout therapy
        - Boxed warning for liver toxicity – LFT monitoring important
- Anticoagulation
    - See DVT/PE section

Bacterial/Viral Eye Infection

Signs/Symptoms/Diagnosis/Complications
- Redness, swelling, inflammation of the eye (Pink Eye)
- Discharge
    - Watery discharge is often associated with viral infection
    - Mucous type discharge is often associated with bacterial infection
- Typically no systemic symptoms
- Adenovirus is most common cause of viral infection
- Bacterial causes are typically
    - Staph, Strep, M. cat, H. flu species

Common Risk Factors
- Immunosuppression
- Lack of tear production which is part of natural defense (dry eyes)
- Contact lenses

Medications to Know
- All topical agents if bacterial infection
    - Erythromycin
    - Polymyxin/trimethoprim
    - Moxifloxacin
    - Sulfacetamide
        - All generally well tolerated other than local effects
        - Systemic effects likely not an issue

Biostatistics Basics

Critical Terms
- Ho = null hypothesis
  - No statistical difference between treatment groups when this is true
- Ha = alternative hypothesis
  - Statistically significant difference between groups when this is true
- P-value of less than 0.05
  - The null hypothesis is rejected and Ha is accepted
- Independent variable
  - Selected by people running the study
- Dependent variables
  - "Depend" upon the independent variables
- Type 1 error – you detected a difference in your study, but a difference in real life doesn't exist
- Type 2 error – you didn't detect a difference in your study and one actually exists
  - Often associated with "power" of a study
  - Benchmark power is usually 80%
- Confidence interval
  - Range of values that you think the "real life" value lies between
- Variables
  - Nominal (or categorical) – no order or number system attached, can you name them to a group
    - I.e. male or female
  - Ordinal - Numbered system, but no sound objective difference between each number
    - I.e. pain scale
  - Continuous – objective, measurable difference between each individual unit
    - Ratio – has an absolute zero (Kelvin temperature)
    - Interval – doesn't have an absolute zero (Celsius temperature)
- Discrete variables
  - Countable, but can't have fractions like you can with continuous variables when measuring
    - I.e. COPD exacerbations/year
- Chi-squared test

- o Often used for nominal data
- T-test
  - o Continuous data
  - o Mean, median, mode apply
  - o "Normal distribution"
  - o Typically only used for one set of data
- Anova
  - o Used for continuous data
  - o Can be used for multiple groups of data
- Sign or Wilcoxon test
  - o Used with ordinal data
- Number Needed to Treat
  - o The number of people treated with an intervention that it takes to see the result or outcome
  - o The higher the NNT, the less likely the outcome desired with the intervention
- Number Needed to Harm
  - o The number of people treated with an intervention that it takes to see the harmful effect
  - o The higher the NNH, the "safer" the intervention likely is
- Study Designs – Descending order in strength of evidence
  - o Randomized controlled trials
  - o Cohort
  - o Case Control studies
  - o Cross Sectional Surveys
  - o Case Study
  - o Expert Opinion
  - o *No consensus on where meta-analysis falls and may depend upon the researcher(s) doing the meta-analysis, but probably toward the upper end of this list (Analysis of multiple different studies on a similar topic)
- Clinical significance
  - o Meaningful benefit to a patient population in clinical practice
- Statistical significance
  - o Evidence of a treatment causing a change
  - o This doesn't necessarily mean that the change is clinically significance

Bipolar Disorder

Signs/Symptoms/Diagnosis/Complications
- Very severe mood swings
- Mania
    - High self-esteem (grandiosity)
    - Way more talkative than normal
    - Constant changing of topics during conversation (racing thoughts)
    - Insomnia or just needing less sleep
    - Interrupts normal life (i.e. work, school, commitments), or others can identify that something is strange
    - Psychosis
- Very depressed stages
- Bipolar 1 – have had manic episode(s)
- Bipolar 2 – haven't had a manic episode
- Risk of suicide
- Often huge social and financial problems
    - Relationships
    - Spending sprees with manic episodes
    - Legal problems
    - Work problems

Common Risk Factors
- Other mental health conditions
    - Substance abuse
    - Anxiety
    - Post-traumatic stress disorder
    - ADHD

Medications to Know
- Mood Stabilizers
    - Lithium
        - Used for acute and maintenance treatment
        - SE's – CNS, ataxia, GI, tremor, hypothyroid, reduce kidney function
        - Toxicity signs – nausea, vomiting, sedation, uncoordinated movements, tremor
        - Coma/seizure risk at very high levels
        - Normal target level 0.5-1.2
        - Notorious drug interactions with common medications (i.e. NSAIDs, thiazide diuretics)
        - TSH, kidney function monitoring important

- Valproic acid
  - Indications; bipolar, seizures, migraines, sometimes used off label for aggressive type behaviors
  - SE's – CNS, GI, and lots of unique, rare side effects (reduced platelets, elevated ammonia, hair loss, LFT elevation)
  - Typical target level 50-100
  - Watch interaction with lamotrigine
  - Multiple dosage forms can have slightly different bioavailability
- Carbamazepine
  - Often used for trigeminal neuralgia, sometimes seizures
  - CNS side effects, GI
  - Induces multiple CYP enzymes – be on the lookout for reduced concentrations of meds that are metabolized via this pathway (lots of common 3A4 interactions)
  - Considered an auto-inducer – can reduce its own levels
  - Levels aren't as important in treating trigeminal neuralgia (unless signs of toxicity)
  - Liver function, CBC, sodium (can cause SIADH) are important monitoring parameters
  - Steven Johnson's syndrome – severe, rare rash is possible
  - Usual target levels 4-12 mcg/mL
- Lamotrigine
  - Sedation, CNS side effects
  - Hallmark RASH side effect – usually when started at too high of a dose or increased too quickly
  - Takes a bit of time (weeks to months) to get to higher doses when titrating appropriately to minimize rash risk
  - Drug interaction with valproic acid (likely need to reduce dose of lamotrigine)
  - Enzyme inducers (i.e. phenytoin, carbamazepine) can reduce concentrations of lamotrigine in the body

- Antidepressants
  - See Depression for breakdown of individual agents
  - Used to help with depressive episodes
  - Can induce mania, especially when used alone
    - Due to this, often given with a mood stabilizer
- Antipsychotics

- See Schizophrenia for individual agents
- Usually an add on to a mood stabilizer if uncontrolled symptoms remain
- Used in treatment of acute mania

BPH

Signs/Symptoms/Diagnosis/Complications
- Overgrowth, or enlargement of the prostate over time
- Incredibly common cause of urinary retention
- Inadequate flow (prostate blocks ureter)
- Frequency
- Patients may strain when urinating
- Incomplete bladder emptying
- Urine dribbling
- UTI's, stones and damage to the bladder and urinary system can result as complications from BPH
- Anticholinergics and alpha agonist activity can exacerbate
- May see an elevation in PSA (Prostate specific antigen)

Common Risk Factors
- Obesity
- Family history
- Age

Medications to Know
- 5-alpha Reductase Inhibitors
    - Finasteride, dutasteride
    - Sexual impairment is primary adverse effect
    - Caution caregivers (younger females) about handling in pregnancy (category X)
    - Takes a long time to begin working - weeks to months
- Alpha-blockers
    - Tamsulosin, terazosin, doxazosin
    - Non-selective alpha blockers can be used for hypertension and BPH (terazosin and doxazosin)
    - Tamsulosin is more selective for the bladder
    - They can work quickly to help relieve symptoms unlike the 5 alpha reductase inhibitors
    - Orthostasis is major risk for these medications
- Anticholinergics
    - Tolterodine, oxybutynin
    - These medications can exacerbate urinary retention, but also can help relieve frequency and other bladder symptoms
    - Use very cautiously in BPH and likely with involvement of specialty (urology)
    - See urinary Incontinence for more information

Cholelithiasis

Signs/Symptoms/Diagnosis/Complications
- Common term: gallstones
- Abdominal pain – usually upper right quadrant
    - Typically quick onset and can get rapidly worse
    - May require intervention
- Fever possible
- Cholesterol component to many gallstones
- Stones can possibly block the bile duct and lead to jaundice

Common Risk Factors
- Age >60
- High cholesterol
- Obesity
- Estrogen replacement therapy
- Diabetes
- More common in females

Medications to Know
- If stone(s) are frequently causing problems, surgical intervention is most common
- Ursodiol
    - Dissolves cholesterol which can be an important component of gallstones
    - GI side effects, CNS possible, dizziness, headache
    - Likely used if surgery is not appropriate or if patient is not a surgical candidate and if felt that cholesterol is a significant component of stones
    - Monitor liver function

Chronic Kidney Disease

Signs/Symptoms/Diagnosis/Complications
- Slow loss or reduction in kidney function over time (years)
- "Creatinine creep" – slow rise in creatinine over time is an indicator of chronic kidney disease
- Kidney function generally declines with age
- At later stages, changes in electrolytes
    - Hyperkalemia can be life threatening if not monitored, addressed
    - Phosphorus accumulation is also important
        - Phosphate binders often used in end stages
- Dialysis in patients with end stage CKD may be necessary
- Accumulation and monitoring of medications that are cleared by the kidney is a vital role for the pharmacist
- Possible signs of CKD
    - Fluid retention
    - Changes in urination
    - Vague symptoms like nausea, fatigue, itching
    - Resistant hypertension
- Increased fracture risk
- Anemia (reduction in erythropoietin production)
- Elevation in Parathyroid Hormone
    - Released in response to low calcium levels

Common Risk Factors
- Diabetes
- Hypertension
- Cardiovascular disease
- Smoking
- Obesity
- African descent, Native American
- Older age

Medications to Know
- Antihypertensives – reduce the pressure on the kidney
- ACE/ARB
    - Delay progression of kidney disease
    - Can induce acute renal failure however, particularly in the setting of renal artery stenosis or use of other meds like NSAIDs, diuretics
- Diuretic therapy

- - Used in the setting of fluid overload
- Anemia management
  - Erythropoietin (ESA's)
  - Usually iron supplementation necessary with ESA use
- Statin therapy
- Phosphate Binders (lowers phosphorus levels in the body)
  - Calcium acetate
    - Administered with meals (possibly snacks)
    - Need to watch calcium levels (contains calcium)
    - GI and hypercalcemia are most common adverse effects
    - Makes sense to use calcium based if hypocalcemia
  - Calcium Carbonate
    - Similar potential problem with elevation in calcium levels
  - Sevelamer
    - Used if elevated calcium level is a problem with calcium acetate
    - Administer with meals
    - GI side effects
  - Aluminum based phosphate binders
    - In general, avoid due to potential toxicity
- Vitamin D analogs
  - Used to help reduce parathyroid hormone
  - Can elevate calcium levels
- Calcimemetics (i.e. cinacalcet)
  - Can reduce parathyroid levels in setting in elevated calcium when vitamin D analogs can worsen the hypercalcemia

Cirrhosis

Signs/Symptoms/Diagnosis/Complications
- Damage/scarring of the liver due to continuous insults; common causes
    - Hepatitis
    - Alcoholism
- May see an elevation in INR (liver makes clotting factors) even in patients not on anticoagulation
- Yellow skin/eyes
- Bruising/bleeding easily
- Swelling/fluid accumulation
    - Particularly in the abdomen (ascites)
    - May also occur in the legs
- Nausea
- Complications
    - Portal hypertension causes enlargement of veins)
    - Esophageal varices (enlarged veins that can rupture) – also remember that cirrhosis can increase the risk of bleed – i.e. thin the blood via reduced clotting factors
    - Enlargement of the spleen
- Alcoholics often will have nutritional deficiencies
    - B12 deficiency
    - Thiamine
- Hepatic encephalopathy
    - Buildup of toxins in the blood due to the liver's inability to break down waste products
    - Ammonia (NH_3) accumulation can cause CNS effects/changes
- Cirrhosis patients at higher risk of;
    - Liver cancer
    - Fractures
- Elevated LFT's especially in early to moderate stages of cirrhosis
    - LFT's may look normal in end stage liver disease as there isn't much more damage that can be done

Common Risk Factors
- Chronic alcohol use
- Hepatitis B or C
- Obesity

Medications to Know
- Treating the underlying cause of cirrhosis is important
    - Alcoholism

- Hepatitis
- Obesity – weight loss
- Portal hypertension and esophageal varices
    - Non-selective beta blocker
- Hepatic encephalopathy – target reducing ammonia levels
    - Lactulose
        - Reduces amount of ammonia potential in the intestine
        - Also rarely used for constipation
        - Aggressiveness of dosing usually depends upon tolerability
        - Adverse effects are GI (diarrhea mostly)
    - Rifaximin
        - Antibiotic
        - Prevents bacteria from producing byproducts that increase the amount of ammonia
        - Very expensive at this time
- Ascites
    - Use of aldosterone antagonist (i.e. spironolactone)
    - May be used in combo with loop diuretics to remove excess fluid from the body
- Supplements as deficiencies are identified
    - B12
    - Folic Acid
    - Thiamine

Clostridium Difficile (C. Diff.)

Signs/Symptoms/Diagnosis/Complications
- Watery diarrhea
- Weight loss
- Cramping
- Dehydration risk
- Potential cause of toxic megacolon
- Spores can live for weeks to potentially months
- Not destroyed by regular alcohol based sanitizers
    - Need to wash hands with soap and water
- Stool testing for diagnosis

Common Risk Factors
- Healthcare associated transmission risk (i.e. long term care, hospitalization)
- Proton Pump Inhibitors
- Frequent/recent antibiotic use (quinolones, clindamycin, etc.)

Medications to Know
- Metronidazole
    - Typical first line especially for mild/moderate outpatient cases
    - See H. Pylori for more info
- Vancomycin
    - One of the only indications you will see ORAL vancomycin used for
    - Poor oral absorption, but not an issue with C. Diff. as infection is within the GI tract
    - GI side effects most common
    - Red man syndrome likely never going to be an issue with oral vancomycin
- Fidaxomicin
    - Refractory cases
    - GI side effects
    - Very expensive
- Probiotics
    - Mixed evidence
    - Can cause GI cramping type side effects
    - Theoretical concern in immunocompromised patients
    - If a patient has recurrent cases of C Diff. providers may be more likely to use them to see if they are helpful

Common Drug Resistant Bacteria

Signs/Symptoms/Diagnosis/Complications
- Methicillin resistant Staph aureus (MRSA)
    o Gram positive
- Pseudomonas Aeruginosa
    o Gram negative
    o Can create a blue-green pigment
- Vancomycin resistant enterococcus (VRE)
    o Gram positive
- Extended Spectrum Beta-Lactamases (ESBL) – typically E. coli, Klebsiella
    o Gram negative

Common Risk Factors
- Overuse, misuse of antibiotics
- Patient specific factors
    o Infection acquired from healthcare institution (i.e. hospital, long term care)
    o Recent, frequent antibiotic use

Medications to Know
- Methicillin resistant Staph aureus (MRSA)
    o Vancomycin, linezolid
    o Doxycycline, sulfamethoxazole/trimethoprim, clindamycin (outpatient possibilities)
    o Avoid penicillin antibiotics
- Pseudomonas Aeruginosa
    o Piperacillin/tazobactam, ceftazidime, ciprofloxacin, levofloxacin
    o Avoid ertapenem
- Vancomycin resistant enterococcus (VRE)
    o Daptomycin, linezolid
    o Avoid vancomycin
- Extended Spectrum Beta-Lactamases (ESBL) – typically E. coli, Klebsiella
    o Penem family (i.e. carbapenem, imipenem)
    o Avoid ceftriaxone, ceftazidime

Congestive Heart Failure

Signs/Symptoms/Diagnosis/Complications
- Inadequate pumping of blood by the heart
- Fatigue and shortness of breath is very common
- Edema (fluid retention) very common in the legs
- Fluid retention also can happen in the abdomen (ascites)
- Coughing
- New York Heart Association Classification
    - Stage – 1 Asymptomatic
    - Stage – 2 Become winded with exertion
    - Stage – 3 Trouble with regular activities
    - Stage – 4 Most severe, symptoms even at rest
- Weight is an important monitoring parameter (rapid increases in weight over a few days can happen in CHF exacerbations)
- Elevations of Pro-BNP (or BNP) a common lab finding during a CHF exacerbation
- Ejection fraction of left ventricle can be suppressed in CHF – usual normal is 55% or higher
- Diuretic therapy often necessary to reduce the amount of fluid in the body
- Narrowing of the arteries, atherosclerosis, hypertension are major contributing factors that can impact hearts pumping ability
- Patients may also present with tachycardia/atrial fibrillation

Common Risk Factors
- Hypertension
- CAD
- MI
- Diabetes
- Valvular heart disease
- Smoking
- Obesity
- Medications that can increase risk of heart failure
    - TZD's (pioglitazone)
    - NSAIDs
    - Pregabalin, gabapentin
    - Calcium Channel blockers

Medications to Know
- Loop diuretics
    - Furosemide, torsemide, bumetanide, ethacrynic acid

- Can dramatically reduce electrolytes
  - Potassium, magnesium, calcium, sodium
- Causes fluid loss thereby helping with symptoms of CHF
- Risk of dehydration (inadequate perfusion of the kidney)
- Monitor kidney function and electrolytes
- Ethacrynic acid you will likely not see used, but its structure does not have a sulfa group, so in patients with significant reactions to all other loops, it may be an option (availability may be an issue however)
- Frequent urination can be a big problem in our elderly patients who may already have frequency and/or incontinence
- Lowers blood pressure, orthostasis concern
* Thiazide like diuretics
  - Metolazone most often used for fluid loss promotion
  - Possibly better efficacy in patients with reduced kidney function versus hydrochlorothiazide
  - May only need to be given periodically (i.e. once or twice per week) in combo with loop diuretic
  - Kidney function, electrolyte monitoring incredibly important especially when used in combo with loops and/or potassium sparing diuretics
* Aldosterone antagonists
  - Spironolactone
    - Heart failure compelling indication
    - See hypertension
* Digoxin
  - Be very careful with hypokalemia risk (increased risk of toxicity/adverse effects) as loops and thiazide like diuretics can cause significant hypokalemia
  - See atrial fibrillation for more info
* ACE Inhibitors, ARBs, Beta-blockers have important compelling indications for heart failure
  - See hypertension
* Statin therapy important for atherosclerosis
* Assessment for antiplatelet therapy is important
* In atrial fibrillation patients with CHF be sure to assess for use of anticoagulation

Constipation

Signs/Symptoms/Diagnosis/Complications
- Difficulty passing bowel movements
- Hard stools
- Straining
- Incomplete evacuation of the bowel
- Risks associated with constipation
    - Obstruction
    - Damage to the colon of intestine
    - Anal fissure

Common Risk Factors
- Older age
- Dehydration
- Physical inactivity
- Use of opioids, anticholinergics, calcium channel blockers, iron supplements, etc.
- Disease states that place patients at risk
    - Parkinson's
    - MS
    - Diabetes
    - Hypothyroidism
    - Stroke

Medications to Know
- Non drug therapy important
    - Hydration
    - Increase fiber intake
    - Physical activity
    - Avoid or minimize contribution from other medications
- Stimulants (i.e. Senokot, bisacodyl)
    - Promote contraction of the bowel
    - Rarely may cause abdominal pain as adverse effect
- Stool softener (i.e. docusate)
    - Help bring in water to the GI tract
    - Usually well tolerated
    - Intended more for the prevention side of things
    - Stimulants and stool softeners often used in combination
        - Especially in patients on opioid therapy
- Osmotics (polyethylene glycol, milk of mag)
    - Draws large amounts of fluid in the GI tract

- - Caution with kidney impairment
    - Usually not an issue with as needed/seldom use
  - Rare risk of magnesium accumulation in kidney disease with frequent use (milk of mag)
- Lubricants (i.e. mineral oil)
  - Avoid due to risk of pneumonitis (aspiration risk)
  - Also can prevent absorption of fat soluble vitamins
- Enema's (i.e. Fleets)
  - Rectal insertion
  - Rare, but serious - can cause electrolyte disturbances especially in patients with CKD
    - Acute phosphate nephropathy
- Lubiprostone
  - Calcium channel activator
  - Nausea is primary adverse effect
  - $$$ expensive treatment option at this time in comparison to other agents

COPD

Signs/Symptoms/Diagnosis/Complications
- COPD characteristics in comparison to asthma
    - Irreversible lung disorder
    - Usually not impacted by triggers
    - Older patients
    - Sputum common
    - Chronic smoking or other environmental long term cause almost always present
- GOLD Guidelines
    - Mild FEV1 >80%
    - Moderate FEV1 50-80%
    - Severe FEV1 30-50%
    - Very Severe <30% or <50% and chronic respiratory failure

Common Risk Factors
- Smoking
- Age
- Long term exposure to smoke/fumes
- Alpha-1-antitrypsan deficiency

Medications to Know
- Short acting beta agonists and/or short acting anticholinergic should be available for acute dyspnea
- Usual controller medication Work Flow: Anticholinergic or LABA -> then Anticholinergic and LABA combination -> add inhaled corticosteroids if frequent exacerbations -> PDE-4 inhibitors -> Theophylline
- Short Acting Anticholinergics
    - Ipratropium
    - Dry mouth
- Long Acting Anticholinergics
    - Tiotropium, aclidinium
    - Dry mouth is common adverse effect
    - Usually don't worry about systemic anticholinergic effects
- Short Acting Beta Agonists
    - Albuterol, levalbuterol
    - See asthma for more information
- Long Acting Beta Agonists
    - Salmeterol, formoterol
    - See asthma section

- Inhaled corticosteroids
    - Fluticasone, Budesonide
    - See asthma section
- PDE-4 inhibitor
    - Roflumilast
    - Oral medication
    - GI side effects
    - Weight loss risk in our frail patients
    - Small risk of psychiatric events
    - 3A4 metabolic pathway, so potential for interactions
- Theophylline
    - See asthma

Coronary Artery Disease

Signs/Symptoms/Diagnosis/Complications
- Blockage or partial blockage of coronary arteries
- Due to atherosclerosis
- Often asymptomatic until an event (i.e. MI)
- Angina (chest pain) is a possibly complication
- Shortness of breath

Common Risk Factors
- Age
- Hypertension
- Smoking
- Males
- Obese
- Diabetes
- Hyperlipidemia
- Physical inactivity

Medications to Know
- Primary focus is going to be on
    - Statin therapy (See hyperlipidemia)
    - Aspirin
        - Adverse effect profile of NSAIDs
        - Not as much concern for kidney/CHF/edema exacerbations with low dose aspirin
        - Platelet inhibition is primary activity so bleed/bruise risk is primary concern
        - Prevents platelet aggregation
        - If patient has past GI bleed history, this will often have to be weighed with past cardiovascular history
        - Enteric coated may help with GI upset
    - Hypertension (See hypertension)
        - Beta-blockers
        - ACE Inhibitors

Crohn's Disease

Signs/Symptoms/Diagnosis/Complications
- Inflammatory disease of the bowel can lead to
    - Ulcers
    - Fistulas
    - Bowel obstruction
- Diarrhea
- Weight loss
- Inflammation can be in different locations of the GI tract (spotty) – surgery utilized, but not curative for the condition which differs from Ulcerative Colitis
- Abdominal pain, cramping
- Blood in stool
- Fever
- Fatigue

Common Risk Factors
- Usually develops at a younger adult age (20's)
- Whites, Jewish descent
- NSAIDs
- Cigarette Smoking

Medications to Know
- Mesalamine
    - GI adverse effects most common
    - Typical first line (or possibly sulfasalazine)
- Sulfasalazine
    - See rheumatoid arthritis
- Corticosteroids
    - Budesonide (Entocort EC)
        - Used to induce remission with an acute flare
        - Typical steroid side effects, but…
            - Maybe has less systemic absorption due to high first pass effect
        - Usually used in shorter term bursts (i.e. a few months)
- Azathioprine
    - GI side effects
    - Immune suppressive (risk of infection)
    - Malignancy risk
    - CBC monitoring, LFT's important to monitor

- - Really important interaction with allopurinol (possibly increases myelosuppressive effects)
- Biologics
  - Infliximab, adalimumab
  - Risk of infection, cancer
  - Common AE's
    - Infusion reaction
    - GI
  - Possible increased LFT's
- Symptom management
  - Psyllium – bulk up stool, try to reduce diarrhea
  - Loperamide – antidiarrheal
  - Acetaminophen – pain (remember to avoid NSAIDs)
  - Chronic bleeding (assess need for iron and B12)

Deep Vein Thrombosis/Pulmonary Embolism

Signs/Symptoms/Diagnosis/Complications
- Pulmonary embolism (PE)
    - Shortness of breath
    - Chest pain
    - Light headed
    - Cough potentially with blood
- Deep Vein Thrombosis (DVT)
    - Redness, swelling, pain in leg
    - One sided
    - Warmth at site
    - Detected by ultrasound
- D-Dimer elevation may be helpful in guiding diagnosis

Common Risk Factors
- Blood clot disorder
    - i.e. Factor V Leiden
- Immobility/prolong bed rest
- Cancer
- Smoking
- Medications
    - Estrogen therapy
    - SERMs
    - Megestrol
- Age
- Family history
- Obesity

Medications to Know
- NOACs (DOACs)
    - Advantages over warfarin – In general;
        - Less drug interactions
        - No monthly INR
        - Fixed dosages
        - Not vitamin k dependent
    - Disadvantages
        - Less experience
        - No lab result to identify adherence issues
        - Some are twice daily
        - Cost

- Shouldn't be used with really poor renal function <15 or <30 depending upon the medication
    - Rivaroxaban
        - Treatment of DVT; 15 mg BID for 21 days – then 20 mg daily
        - Post op prophylaxis 10 mg daily
        - DVT prevention 20 mg daily
        - Afib – 20 mg daily (may reduce to 15 mg daily for reduced kidney function)
        - CrCl <30 don't use
        - Convert from warfarin – DC warfarin when INR is <3 and start rivaroxaban
        - Bleed risk is major adverse effect
        - Major interaction (strong 3A4 inducers, i.e. rifampin can reduce effectiveness)
        - Erythromycin, clarithromycin can increase concentrations
    - Apixaban
        - DVT/PE 10 mg twice daily for 5 days followed by 5 mg twice daily
        - Post op – 2.5 mg BID
        - Afib – 5 mg twice daily
            - Unless patient has 2 of 3: Remember 80, 60, 1.5 – age >80, weight <60 kg, and creatinine >1.5 then 2.5 mg BID
        - Conversion from warfarin (DC warfarin when INR less than 2 and start apixaban)
    - Dabigatran
        - Downsides – twice daily
        - GI bleed risk in patients >75
            - Seems to have fallen out of favor because of this risk
- Warfarin
    - Usual starting dose 1-5 mg (based on clinical experience, current medications, liver failure, age, etc.)
    - Notorious causes of drug interactions and variable INR's
        - Dietary changes of vitamin K
        - Displacement from protein
            - Lot of meds, also malnutrition
        - 2C9 is usually the biggest effect, 3A4 also important
            - Metronidazole, Bactrim (2C9)
        - 3A4 effect

- - - Inhibitors raise INR (i.e. erythromycin, amiodarone etc.)
      - Inducers lower INR (i.e. St. John's Wort)
    - Typically check INR within 2-5 days after initiating a drug that is known to interact with warfarin
    - Impact on bacterial vitamin K production
      - Antibiotics
    - Bleed risk
      - Antiplatelets, NSAIDs (GI bleed especially)
  - Typical goal INR is 2-3
    - Exception; high risk of bleed/falls – clinical judgement for lower value
    - Valve replacement (2.5-3.5)
  - Rare purple toe syndrome (don't load warfarin)
  - Vitamin K is reversal agent – does take some time to work (hours)
- Enoxaparin
  - Injection is the big downside
  - DVT Prophylaxis
    - Usually 40 mg daily or possibly 30 mg BID (twice daily injection is a downside)
    - CrCl less than 30 – 30 mg daily
  - Treatment
    - 1 mg/kg/dose (twice daily)
    - OR 1.5 mg/kg/day once daily
  - Careful in patients who have a history of heparin induced thrombocytopenia (HIT)
  - Rarely may contribute to hyperkalemia
  - Bleed risk is most common adverse effect
  - If bridging to warfarin, discontinue when INR hits target range (usually 2-3)

Delirium

Signs/Symptoms/Diagnosis/Complications
- Confusion
- Anger
- Altered consciousness
- Rambling or incoherent speaking
- Yelling
- Combative, aggressive behavior
- Rapid, unpredictable mood swings
- Withdrawn, inattentive
- Onset is relatively quick
- Lasts hours to weeks, maybe up to a month or two
- Post op (pain and lingering medications)
- Examples of causes
    - Pain
    - Infection
    - Medication
    - Toxins
        - Drug intoxication (i.e. alcohol, illicit drug use)
- Classic medication causes
    - Anticholinergics
        - Sleepers (doxepin, diphenhydramine)
        - Older antihistamines (i.e. diphenhydramine)
        - Cyclobenzaprine
    - Benzodiazepines or Z-drugs for sleep
    - Opioids
    - Drugs with dopamine activity (i.e. carbidopa/levodopa)

Common Risk Factors
- Sensory defects
    - Hearing
    - Visual
- Previous history of delirium
- Older age
- Brain disorders (i.e. dementia)
- Numerous condition

Medications to Know
- Primary goal is identifying and treating what is causing delirium, also comforting patient
    - Discontinue medications that may be contributing

- - - Offer food/drink
    - Assess possible nutritional deficiencies
    - Avoidance of bothersome environmental factors
      - Excessive tubes
      - Physical restraints
      - Bright lights, loud noises etc.
    - Treat pain
    - Addressing incontinence
    - Involve family, familiar caregivers
- When non-drug interventions fail and significant symptoms remain that are putting the patient or others at risk
  - Haloperidol
    - Most experience, studied
    - High EPS – really careful use in Parkinson's patients
  - Atypical antipsychotics
    - Typically less side effects than older haloperidol
    - Less experience/evidence
    - Examples: quetiapine, olanzapine, risperidone
      - Medication with injectable dosage form may be necessary depending upon the situation
  - Clinicians may prefer either agent based upon experience/situation
  - Benzodiazepines
    - Mixed evidence
    - Possible disinhibition (remember they can contribute to delirium)
  - Anticholinergics (i.e. hydroxyzine)
    - Generally avoid
- Any medication used for delirium should have a plan in place to reduce and discontinue as delirium is a short term condition
- Physical restraints should not be used unless no other alternative exists

Dementia

Signs/Symptoms/Diagnosis/Complications
- Symptoms/Signs
    - Memory loss
    - Changes in mood/behavior
        - Aggression
        - Withdrawn
        - Depression
        - Anxiety
        - Hallucination/paranoia
        - Inappropriate behavior
- 3 Really common causes
    - Alzheimer's
        - Plaque's in the brain
        - Most common form of dementia
    - Vascular
        - Loss of blood supply to certain regions of the brain
        - Damaged vessels - Stroke, atherosclerosis can contribute
    - Lewy Body
        - Usually associated with Parkinson's
        - Abnormal clumps of protein found in the brain
- Don't confuse dementia with delirium
    - Delirium is a reversible condition whereas dementia is not
- Rare causes – Huntington's, Traumatic Brain Injury
- Memory loss complications
    - Malnutrition
    - Dehydration
    - Inability to do activities of daily living (ADL's)
        - I.e. bathing, dressing, brushing teeth etc.
    - Safety concerns
        - I.e. driving, cooking etc.
- Risk of aspiration pneumonia (chewing, swallowing implications)
- Mini mental status exam (MMSE)
    - Scored 0-30
    - Higher the better
    - 25-30 (no cognitive impairment)
    - 20-25 (mild)
    - 10-20 (moderate)
    - 0-10 (severe)

Common Risk Factors
- Age
- Diabetes
- Smoking
- Alcoholism
- Family history
- Down syndrome

Medications to Know
- Rule out B12 deficiency, thyroid issues, and possible medication(s), environmental factors contributing to memory loss
- No medication reverses dementia
- Acetylcholinesterase inhibitors
    - Donepezil, rivastigmine, galantamine
    - Used in mild to moderate dementia
    - GI side effects are most common (think opposite effects of anticholinergic medications)
        - Diarrhea, nausea, vomiting
        - Weight loss
    - Rarely can cause insomnia
        - Donepezil is dosed at night in case patient gets GI side effects
            - Can take in the morning if insomnia side effects
    - Rivastigmine comes in a patch formulation
        - Possibly less GI side effects
        - Rarely used due to cost $$$
        - Oral tablets are dosed twice daily
    - Interaction with anticholinergics (they can cause confusion and blunt effects of acetylcholinesterase inhibitors)
- NMDA Antagonist
    - Memantine
    - CNS side effects
    - Used in moderate to severe dementia
    - Dose adjusted with reduced kidney function
    - Can be used in combo with acetylcholinesterase inhibitor
    - 28 mg of XR is approximately equivalent to 20 mg of immediate release

Dementia Related Behaviors

Signs/Symptoms/Diagnosis/Complications
- Patient with dementia may have numerous different behaviors
    - Yelling
    - Anger
    - Physical aggression (hitting, kicking, pinching etc.)
    - Paranoid
    - Hallucinations
    - Anxiety
    - Depression
    - Sexual inappropriateness
    - Repetitive questions/statements
    - Wandering
    - Insomnia

Common Risk Factors
- See risk factors for development of dementia

Medications to Know
- Primary goal; identification of behavior and recognizing that a medication should be your last line therapy of choice
- Questions that need to be asked with behavioral symptoms
    - What happened just before it started?
    - Is there a new medical problem?
    - Are there medications that are causing this new behavior?
    - Are the patient's needs met?
        - Is the person in pain?
        - Hungry?
        - Thirsty?
        - Have to go to the bathroom?
    - Is there an environmental factor or change that is bothering them?
- Medications should only be considered when all non-drug options have been exhausted
- Only use medications for behaviors that are harmful to the patient or placing caregivers or other person's health at risk
    - i.e. If patient has hallucinations and they are not harmful or distressing, you shouldn't need to treat this with medication
- Poor clinical evidence of effectiveness for any of these agents used in dementia
- Antipsychotics

- o Black box warning for increased risk of death in dementia patients
- o Used off label in dementia
  - ▪ Only use for severe, distressing symptoms (aggression, paranoia, hallucinations, delusions)
- Benzodiazepines
  - o Can help with insomnia and anxiety symptoms, but lots of problems with side effects in the elderly
  - o Fall risk
  - o Can exacerbate patient's confusion
  - o Disinhibition is a possible effect (i.e. it may make patients behaviors worse)
- Antidepressants
  - o May help if they have depression
  - o If OCD, anxiety and PTSD history, they may be helpful as well
- Mood stabilizers
  - o Some clinicians will use these medications to help with anger/aggressive behaviors
    - ▪ i.e. valproic acid, lamotrigine

Depression

Signs/Symptoms/Diagnosis/Complications
- Feeling sad
- Loss of interest in things that used to be enjoyable
- Changes in behavior
- Loss of self-esteem
- Changes in sleep pattern
- Changes in eating (loss of appetite or increased eating)
- Risk of suicide
- Common differential diagnosis: Hypothyroid, anemia, fibromyalgia
- PHQ-9 and HAM-D are examples of assessments

Common Risk Factors
- Other mental health conditions
  - PTSD
  - Anxiety
  - Eating disorders
- Family history
- Traumatic events
- Drug abuse
- Chronic illness (cancer, stroke)

Medications to Know
- Important education point to patients that it may take weeks to months for these medications to begin working
- Selection usually based upon adverse effect profile/provider preference
- SSRI's
  - Sertraline, citalopram, escitalopram, fluoxetine, paroxetine
  - Typical first line antidepressant
  - Sexual dysfunction
  - Possibility of hyponatremia (look out for patients already on diuretics)
  - Sertraline most serotonergic – highest risk of loose stools
  - Fluoxetine a little more activating
  - Fluoxetine longest half life
  - Paroxetine a little more sedating, also mild anticholinergic effects – but not nearly as problematic as TCA's
  - Fluvoxamine rarely used due to drug interactions (3A4)
  - Citalopram max of 20 mg in elderly and on commonly used omeprazole (QTc prolongation risk)
- SNRI's

- o Venlafaxine, duloxetine
- o Often used if corresponding pain syndromes (i.e. neuropathy)
- o Venlafaxine typically needs to be used at higher doses for pain benefit
- o Risk of raising blood pressure, especially at higher doses
- o Sexual dysfunction
- Mirtazapine
  - o Sedating (can help with insomnia, particularly at lower doses)
  - o Weight gain – can help with frail elderly with depression
    - Can be a negative in already overweight patients
  - o Option for patients looking to minimize risk of sexual dysfunction side effect
- TCA's
  - o Nortriptyline, amitriptyline
  - o Not first line due to anticholinergic and risk of cardiac issues in attempted suicide through overdose
  - o Highly anticholinergic
    - Dry eyes, mouth, constipation, falls, confusion
  - o Nortriptyline possibly a little more tolerable in the elderly
  - o QTC prolongation risk when in combo with other meds or in high risk patients
  - o Sexual dysfunction
- Trazodone, nefazodone
  - o Nefazodone rarely used due to hepatotoxicity
  - o Trazodone more often used for its sedative properties at low doses
    - 12.5 – 100mg at night
  - o Antidepressant target doses for trazodone are usually higher
  - o Dry mouth, sedation, orthostasis risk
- Bupropion
  - o Activating
  - o Increases the risk of seizures (avoid use)
  - o Can be used for smoking cessation
  - o Option for patients looking to avoid sexual dysfunction adverse effect
- MAOI's
  - o Last line agent
  - o Tyramine - food interaction
  - o Multiple contraindicated drug interactions (i.e. Triptans, SSRI's)

Dysphagia

Signs/Symptoms/Diagnosis/Complications
- Difficulty or painful swallowing
    - Impact on drinking, eating
    - Possible weight loss
- Coughing, gagging
- Regurgitation
- Requiring smaller, cut up foods
- Heartburn may be contributing factor
- Possible causes
    - Damage or scar tissue from stomach acid
    - Esophageal stricture (narrowing of the esophagus)
    - Foreign body
    - Radiation leading to inflammation and damage
    - Esophageal tumor
    - Stroke
    - Parkinson's disorder
- Complications are malnutrition and possible aspiration into the lungs

Common Risk Factors
- Age
- Neurological disorders (i.e. stroke, Parkinson's)

Medications to Know
- For dysphagia caused or exacerbated by GERD/stomach acid
    - PPI's
    - H2 blockers
- Significant dysphagia can lead to
    - Liquid type diets
    - Tube feedings
- Tube feeding administration pearls
    - Keep an eye out for binding interactions
        - Levothyroxine
        - Phenytoin
        - Warfarin
        - Quinolones
    - Interaction with phenytoin and tube feedings
        - Hold feedings for 1-2 hours before/after giving dose of phenytoin
        - If feedings cannot be held, dose of phenytoin will likely need to be increased

- Warfarin
    - Adjust dose to INR, check INR frequently upon initiation/changes in tube feeding
- Quinolones
    - Hold feedings 1 hour before and 2 hours after or increase dose

Essential Tremor

Signs/Symptoms/Diagnosis/Complications
- Rhythmic movement/shaking at a consistent, relatively fast frequency
- Involuntary movement
- Typically starts one sided and often in the hand
- Make sure to identify possible medications that can exacerbate or cause tremor
    - Too much levothyroxine
    - CNS stimulants
    - Beta agonists
    - Caffeine
    - Lithium
    - Antiseizure medications (rarely)
    - SSRI's (rarely)
- Greatly impact ADLs and safety concerns

Common Risk Factors
- Family history
- Elderly

Medications to Know
- All drugs for essential tremor do not have a good side effect profile for our elderly patients, but are often used in relatively low doses
- Beta-blockers
    - See hypertension for more information
    - Typically non-selectives are used for tremor (i.e. propranolol, nadolol)
- Primidone
    - Converted to phenobarbital
    - Historically an old antiseizure medication
    - Sedation, confusion, CNS adverse effects
    - If concerned about toxicity can check primidone and phenobarbital levels
    - Levels aren't routinely checked for tremor if patient is not having signs of toxicity
- Benzodiazepines
    - See anxiety

Failure to Thrive

Signs/Symptoms/Diagnosis/Complications
- Decreased appetite
- Weight loss
- Physical inactivity
- Malnutrition
- Frailty

Common Risk Factors
- Numerous chronic medical condition associated with failure to thrive (a few common ones)
    - Cancer
    - Depression
    - CHF
    - COPD
    - Stroke
- Common medications associated with failure to thrive
    - Anticholinergics
    - Beta-blockers
    - Opioids
    - Benzodiazepines

Medications to Know
- No medication to treat failure to thrive
- Management
    - Treat underlying disease states
    - Avoid/minimize medications that may be contributing
    - Identify potential differential diagnosis; for example
        - Thyroid changes
        - Anemia
        - Psych evaluation
        - Metabolic abnormalities
        - Medication toxicity

Falls in the Elderly

Signs/Symptoms/Diagnosis/Complications
- Frequent cause of injury
    - Fracture
    - Bleed/bruising
    - Traumatic brain injury
- Physical Contributors
    - Weakness
    - Gait
    - Balance
    - Orthostasis
    - Vision
    - Cognition
- Environmental considerations
    - Poor lighting
    - Hazardous object in hallways etc.
    - Bathroom/bedroom conditions
    - Avoiding steps
    - Support rails as appropriate

Common Risk Factors
- History of falls
- >85
- Multiple diagnosis
    - Dementia
    - Arthritis
    - Stroke
    - Neuropathy
    - Anemia
    - Vitamin D deficiency
- Polypharmacy
- Use of
    - Sedatives/hypnotics
    - Anticholinergics
    - Diuretics
    - Antihypertensives

Medications to Know
- Reduce/minimize high risk medications as above
- Correlate timing of new medications to new onset of falls
- May have relaxed goals

- - Hypertension
  - Diabetes (avoid risk of hypoglycemia)
- For those with injury/fractures
  - Treat pain (acetaminophen first line)
  - Opioids can be utilized with close monitoring
  - NSAIDs get a little challenging to use with many elderly on anticoagulants, have CHF, kidney disease
- Address possible deficiencies
  - Vitamin D
  - Anemia (due to B12, iron, etc.)

Generalized Anxiety Disorder

Signs/Symptoms/Diagnosis/Complications
- Fear or anxiety
- Loss of control over natural situations that cause stress/anxiety
- Tachycardia, increased BP, trembling, GI upset, rapid breathing
- May include many different subtypes
    - Social anxiety disorder
    - Panic attacks
    - Fear of specific things
- Anxiety may be associated with other conditions
    - Pain
    - Hyperthyroidism
    - Drug withdrawal
    - Respiratory issues (i.e. COPD)

Common Risk Factors
- Drugs/alcohol
- Family history
- Comorbid mental illness
- Trauma/acute stress

Medications to Know
- Be sure that medical causes of anxiety are ruled out and addressed prior to considering pharmacotherapy
- Psychotherapy should always be a strong consideration
- Buspirone
    - Advantages
        - Non-controlled substance
        - Pretty well tolerated (even in older patients) compared to benzodiazepines
    - Disadvantage
        - Takes a while to work
- SSRI's
    - Frequently used for anxiety
    - Still usually take a while to work in anxiety as well as depression
    - See depression for pearls on individual agents/class
- Benzodiazepines
    - Lorazepam, clonazepam, diazepam
    - Side effects, similar to alcohol in a pill
    - Sedation

- Slurred speech
- Confusion
- Fall risk
- Remember "LOT" lorazepam, oxazepam, temazepam – less likely to accumulate in the elderly
- Flumazenil is reversal agent
- Other antidepressants
  - SNRI's
  - Mirtazapine
  - Trazodone
  - Bupropion

GERD

Signs/Symptoms/Diagnosis/Complications
- Epigastric pain
  - Contents of the stomach (acid) into the esophagus
- Regurgitation
- Chest pain
- Sore/hoarse throat
- Foreign object sensations in the throat
- In elderly, may see atypical signs (i.e. dry cough)
- Classic medications that exacerbate GERD
  - NSAIDs
  - Corticosteroids
  - Bisphosphonates
- Complications
  - Barrett's Esophagus – alteration in the cells to a pre-cancerous state
  - Esophageal bleeding/ulceration
  - Stricture (narrowing) of the esophagus
- Non-pharmacologic options
  - Avoid trigger foods (i.e. spicy, chocolate etc.)
  - Tight clothing
  - Weight loss
  - Frequent, smaller meals
  - Avoiding lying down after eating
  - Elevating the head of the bed

Common Risk Factors
- Obesity
- Smoking
- Asthma
- Gastroparesis
- Diabetes
- Hiatal hernia

Medications to Know
- Antacids (i.e. calcium carbonate)
  - Identify patients with frequent use as they should possibly be on strong acid suppressing agents
  - Hypercalcemia (rare, likely only with frequent use)
  - Binding interactions common
    - Quinolones

- - - Tetracycline antibiotics
    - Levothyroxine
  - Constipation
- H2 blockers (i.e. ranitidine, famotidine)
  - Keep an eye out for dose adjustments in CKD
  - Possible accumulation leading to CNS problems (rare, but more likely in CKD)
  - Not quite as potent as PPI's
  - Avoid cimetidine in the elderly due to numerous drug interactions via 3A4
- PPI's (i.e. omeprazole, pantoprazole)
  - Most potent acid blocker
  - Generally dosed 30 minutes before a meal for maximal effect
  - May take a few days for max effect
  - Osteoporosis risk
  - B12 and magnesium deficiency possible
  - Trend toward increasing C. diff risk
  - Notable interactions with omeprazole
    - Citalopram max 20 mg daily
    - Clopidogrel (controversial how clinically significant)
  - May see twice daily dosing for refractory cases of GERD
  - Also may see PPI in the morning in combo with H2 blocker at night
  - Try to treat GERD for 4-8 weeks and reassess use due to some of the longer term risks
  - Often PPI's get started in a hospital stay and get left on board, make sure they are frequently reassessed
  - Higher risk situations like Barrett's, NSAID or corticosteroid use will more likely require long term use
- Sucralfate
  - Frequent dosing bothersome for some patients (usually TID or QID)
  - Binding interactions possible
    - Administer other meds 2 hours before giving sucralfate
    - i.e. levothyroxine, warfarin

Geriatric Vaccines

Pneumococcal 13 Valent Conjugate Vaccine
- One time lifetime dose
- Injection
- Inactive (non-living)
- 1 year separation from Pneumococcal Polysaccharide 23 valent
- Indicated for everyone over age of 65

Pneumococcal Polysaccharide 23 Valent Vaccine
- Up to 3 lifetime doses (only 1 after the age of 65)
- Injection
- Inactive
- Indicated for all patients 65 and older
- If received before age 65, need to wait 5 years
    - I.e. - If given at age 63, do not give until patient is 68
- If neither PPSV 23 or PCV 13 have been given at age 65, give PCV 13
    - Then wait 1 year and give PPSV 23

Zoster Live Vaccine (Zostavax)
- One time dose
- Injection
- Live vaccine
- Special freezer requirements
- Peak incidence of Shingles around age 60
- Indicated as early as age 50, but typically given between 60-64
- Effectiveness wanes as patients age, more studies of effectiveness in >70 y/o may be coming

Influenza Vaccine
- Inactivated vaccine
- Injection
- Given annually
- High dose available, ACIP does not take a stance yet on recommending high dose or not
    - A little more expensive
    - Many clinicians are using it for all >65
    - Some are reserving for higher risk populations (i.e. smokers, lung disease etc.)
- Do not use nasal influenza vaccine
- Typically takes 2 weeks to form antibodies
- Start giving vaccine in October timeframe

- Give vaccine until influenza is no longer circulating
  - Usually April-May timeframe

Glaucoma

Signs/Symptoms/Diagnosis/Complications
- Elevation in eye pressure
- Damage to the optic nerve due to that pressure
- Loss in peripheral vision
- #1 cause of blindness
- Damage not reversible
- Acute angle closure glaucoma
    - "closed angle"
    - Rapid changes
    - Severe headache
    - Eye pain
    - Not common
- Open angle glaucoma
    - Very common
    - Increase in pressure slowly which causes damage
    - Classic glaucoma medications utilized

Common Risk Factors
- Increased intraocular pressure
- Age > 60
- Family history
- Diabetes, hypertension
- Chronic topical (eye) corticosteroid use

Medications to Know
- Goal is to reduce intraocular pressure and prevent/delay further damage
- Prostaglandins
    - i.e. latanoprost
    - Side effects
        - eye pigment changes
        - eye irritation
- Beta-blockers
    - i.e. timolol
    - Systemic side effects rare but possible
        - Bradycardia, hypotension etc.
- Alpha agonist
    - i.e. brimonidine
    - Increases outflow, decreases production of aqueous humor
    - Eye irritation

- Carbonic anhydrase inhibitor
    - i.e. dorzolamide
    - Can leave a metallic taste in the mouth
    - Oral option sometimes used in refractory cases – can have impact on electrolytes/kidney function
- Cholinergic agonist
    - i.e. pilocarpine
    - Miosis (pinpoint pupil)
    - Blurry vision

Gout

Signs/Symptoms/Diagnosis/Complications
- Classic symptom; severe pain in the big toe
- Redness, warmth, painful, swollen joint(s)
- Often at night
- Formation of urate crystals contributed by elevated uric acid
- Ballpark normal uric acid levels (2.5-6)
    - Generally elevated in gout
- Urate crystals can form and cause kidney stones
- Tophi
    - Nodules at a joint or joint(s) because of crystallized urate deposits
    - Usually develop over longer periods of time
    - Can impact joint function
    - Generally more painful during a gout attack
- Onset usually middle aged (30-50)

Common Risk Factors
- Alcohol use
- Metabolic disease/obesity
- Seafood (foods high in purines)
- Family history
- Males more common than females

Medications to Know
- Allopurinol
    - Side effects – rash, GI
    - Dose adjust with worsening kidney function
    - Used for PREVENTION, reduction of uric acid, NOT for acute treatment of a gout attack
    - Reduces production of uric acid in the body
- Colchicine
    - Dose limiting side effect is most often diarrhea (high percentage of patients)
    - Dose adjustments in CKD
    - Can be used for both treatment and prevention
- NSAIDs
    - Used for acute management of pain associated with a gout flare
    - Often will see indomethacin preferentially used by providers, but doesn't have to be

- ▪ Indomethacin does have a high incidence of GI side effects
  - • Possibly will see GI protection used with it
- ▪ See osteoarthritis for more clinical information on NSAIDs
- Corticosteroids
  - Acute flare management only
  - Alternative to patients intolerable to NSAIDs or who have contraindications
  - See rheumatoid arthritis for more clinical information
- Febuxostat
  - Similar mechanism as allopurinol
  - Meant for prophylaxis
  - More expensive than allopurinol, but alternative if allopurinol ineffective/intolerable
- Probenecid
  - Removal of uric acid in the body by increasing kidney excretion
  - GI upset adverse effect
  - Some drug interactions with other kidney cleared medications
  - Need adequate kidney function for the medication to work

Headaches

Signs/Symptoms/Diagnosis/Complications
- Tension
    - Generalized, mild to moderate pain
    - Most common
    - Non-drug and medication treatments can be effective
    - Chronic >15 days per year
- Migraine
    - Nausea and vomiting can be associated
    - Visual disturbances are possible (aura)
    - Generally one sided
    - Severity and length can vary greatly between patients
    - Often incredibly sensitive to noise, light, and possibly smells
- Cluster
    - Incredibly painful
    - Usually multiple attacks for a period of time (weeks), then a headache free period
- Rebound headaches or medication overuse headaches
    - Headaches come back when medication has been stopped
    - Important to educate patients to not use acute medications chronically and/or use appropriate prophylaxis agents to prevent overuse

Common Risk Factors
- Stress
- Family history
- Environmental factors
- Males (cluster)
- Onset usually in younger patients, but can continue later on in life

Medications to Know
- Tension
    - Acetaminophen generally safest in the elderly
    - NSAIDs are alternative option but can be riskier if used chronically
    - Caffeine containing medications may also be considered
        - Frequent use can raise blood pressure, pulse
    - Triptans can be utilized, but usually not needed
- Migraine
    - Acetaminophen/NSAIDs can be used for mild to moderate
    - Triptans

- Adverse effects – CNS changes, dizziness
- Meant for acute relief, not prophylaxis
- Can be used in combination with NSAIDs or acetaminophen
- Potential for serotonin interactions (SSRI's, tramadol etc.)
            - Prevention
                - Topiramate
                    - Cognitive slowing
                    - Sedation
                - Beta-blockers – see hypertension
                - Valproic Acid – see bipolar disorder
                    - Typically don't worry about drug levels unless toxicity
                - TCA's – see depression
    - Cluster
        - Oxygen
        - Triptans
        - Prevention
            - Calcium channel blockers first line (non-DHP)
    - Rebound headaches common causes
        - Caffeine containing compounds
        - Butalbital
        - Opioids
        - Triptans
        - Simple analgesics (APAP, NSAIDs)

HIV/AIDS

Signs/Symptoms/Diagnosis/Complications
- Suppresses the immune system
- At risk for opportunistic infections
- Sexually or blood borne transmission
- Defined as AIDS when CD4 count drops below 200 or have an AIDS defining illness
- Common opportunistic infections
    - Pneumocystis carinii pneumonia (PCP)
    - Cytomegalovirus (CMV)
    - Tuberculosis (TB)
    - Candidiasis
    - Toxoplasmosis
    - Cryptococcus meningitis
    - Kaposi's sarcoma
- Complications
    - Can cause dementia type symptoms
    - Kidney disease
    - Wasting disease
    - Rapid mutations in virus makes adherence incredibly important

Common Risk Factors
- Typically transmission is not going to happen in our geriatric population
- Unprotected sex
- IV drug users
- Co-infection with another STD

Medications to Know
- Non-Nucleoside Reverse Transcriptase Inhibitors (efavirenz, delaviridine, etravirine)
    - CNS side effects, psychiatric changes
        - Hallucinations, abnormal dreams etc.
    - Hepatotoxic
    - Rash – can monitor if mild, but DC if severe
    - Potentially lowers seizure threshold
- Protease Inhibitors (atazanavir, lopinavir/ritonavir, saquinavir)
    - "Buffalo hump" – fat redistribution
    - Elevates blood sugars
    - Tons of drug interactions through 3A4

- Nucleotide Reverse Transcriptase Inhibitor (tenofovir)
  - Lactic acidosis/fatty liver boxed warning
  - May exacerbate osteoporosis
  - GI adverse effects
  - Elevation in cholesterol
- PCP – treatment Bactrim
- CMV – ganciclovir or valgangciclovir
- TB – see TB
- Candidiasis – fluconazole
  - Notorious for drug interactions via CYP3A4
- Toxoplasmosis – pyrimethamine
- Cryptococcus – Ampho B, flucytosine, fluconazole

Hyperlipidemia

Signs/Symptoms/Diagnosis/Complications
- Asymptomatic
- Intensity of statin therapy is determined by risk factors
- Triglycerides is primary target if >500
    - Risk of pancreatitis if elevated triglycerides
- Elevated LDL
- Buildup of plaque contributing to MI, stroke, etc.

Common Risk Factors
- Important factors that go into CV risk calculation
    - Diabetes
    - Hypertension
    - Age
    - Smoking
    - Cholesterol levels
    - CVD (Peripheral vascular disease, CHF, CAD)
    - Blood pressure
- LDL > 190 recommended high intensity statin

Medications to Know
- High Intensity (approximately >50% reduction in LDL)
    - Rosuvastatin 20-40 mg daily
    - Atorvastatin 40-80 mg daily
- Moderate intensity (30-50% reduction in LDL)
    - Rosuvastatin 5-10 mg daily
    - Atorvastatin 10-20 mg daily
    - Simvastatin 20-40 mg daily (in general, avoid 80 mg/day)
    - Pravastatin 40-80 mg daily
    - Lovastatin 40 mg daily
- Low Intensity (<30% reduction in LDL)
    - Simvastatin 10 mg daily
    - Pravastatin 10-20 mg daily
    - Lovastatin 20 mg daily
- ALL Statins
    - Myopathy risk
    - Rhabdomyolysis (rare, but severe)
        - Elevated CPK
        - Risk of renal failure
        - Fibrates can increase risk
- Atorvastatin

- o No preference on dosing at night
- o Major metabolism through 3A4
- Rosuvastatin
  - o Most common "highest" intensity statin
  - o Generic in 2016
- Simvastatin
  - o A few common interactions to adjust dosing (amlodipine, diltiazem, verapamil, amiodarone)
  - o Manufacturer recommends evening dosing
- Lovastatin
  - o Major pathway 3A4
- Pravastatin
  - o Multiple pathways for metabolism
- Gemfibrozil
  - o Increases risk of rhabdomyolysis when used with statins
  - o GI adverse effects
  - o Targets triglycerides
- Fenofibrate
  - o Possible increase in rhabdomyolysis with statins, usually less risk then gemfibrozil
  - o Target is to reduce triglycerides
- Niacin
  - o Target triglycerides
  - o Possible increase in HDL
  - o Flushing adverse effect, can take with aspirin to minimize, but obviously must be aware of aspirin adverse effect profile/risks
  - o Can increase uric acid (gout)

Hypertension

Signs/Symptoms/Diagnosis/Complications
- Typically Asymptomatic
- Increased risk of stroke, MI, kidney disease, visual problems, heart failure, aneurysm, metabolic syndrome
- JNC-8
    - Less than 60 y/o, or CKD, or diabetes – goal <140/90
    - >60 y/o – goal <150/90

Common Risk Factors
- Obese
- Sodium intake
- Tobacco
- Family history
- Blacks
- Age
- Inactivity
- Excessive alcohol
- Drug induced hypertension
    - Pseudoephedrine
    - Stimulants
    - NSAIDs
    - ESA's
    - Mirabegron
    - Caffeine
    - Estrogen
    - SNRI's (usually at higher doses)

Medications to Know
- ACE Inhibitors
    - Cough
    - Hyperkalemia
    - Angioedema (very rare, but very serious)
    - Major compelling indications (diabetes, CKD, stroke, CHF, MI)
    - Monitor kidney function/potassium
    - 30% increase in creatinine is concerning following initiating/increase
    - Less effective in blacks
    - ALL blood pressure reducing medications can cause orthostasis

- ARBs
    - Think ACE Inhibitors with less cough
    - Avoid using ACE and ARBs together
- Thiazide diuretics (chlorthalidone and hydrochlorothiazide)
    - Major compelling indications (CHF or edema, stroke reduction)
    - Elevates uric acid (risk for gout flares)
    - Frequent urination (dose earlier in the day)
    - Risk of dehydration
    - Monitor kidney function and electrolytes
    - Cause/worsen erectile dysfunction
    - Elevates blood sugars (typically not clinically significant at low doses)
- Beta-blockers
    - Selectivity is important
    - Metoprolol and atenolol are classic beta-1 selective
    - Propranolol, nadolol are classic non-selective (beta-1 and beta-2 activity)
    - Carvedilol and labetalol have some alpha activity
    - Compelling Indications: Angina, CHF (stable), Post MI, Atrial fibrillation
    - Avoid abruptly stopping unless very serious adverse effect
    - Side effects
        - Sedation/fatigue
        - Low pulse
        - Increase asthma exacerbation risk or block beta-2 agonists effectively, more of an issue with non-selective
        - Mask hypoglycemia (most should still sweat) – non-selective beta-blocker usually higher concern
        - Exacerbate erectile dysfunction
    - Propranolol often used in:
        - Migraine
        - Esophageal Varices (portal hypertension associated with cirrhosis)
        - Essential Tremor
- Calcium Channel Blockers
    - Non-Dihydropyridines
        - Verapamil, Diltiazem
        - Act on heart and vessels
        - Can be used for rate control in atrial fibrillation
        - Monitor pulse

- - -
      - Watch for interactions via CYP3A4 inhibition
      - Edema, constipation major side effects
    - Dihydropyridines
      - Amlodipine, nifedipine
      - Compelling indications; Raynaud's, angina
      - Edema, orthostasis (ALL meds that lower blood pressure can cause orthostasis)
- Central Acting Alpha-2 agonists
  - Clonidine, methyldopa, Guanfacine
  - Not first line for hypertension
  - Drowsiness, dizziness, dry mouth (avoid in elderly if possible)
  - May see used for psych disorders occasionally (ADHD etc.)
  - Clonidine is used for opioid withdrawal symptom management
  - Rebound hypertension troublesome if stopped abruptly
- Direct Acting Vasodilators
  - Hydralazine, minoxidil
  - Hydralazine can exacerbate/contribute to Lupus type symptoms
  - Hydralazine dosed frequently which can be a pain for adherence
  - Minoxidil used for hair loss (alopecia)
  - May see hydralazine/nitrate combination in heart failure for blacks as ACE/ARBs may not be as effective in that population
- Aldosterone Receptor Antagonists
  - Eplerenone, spironolactone
  - Hyperkalemia, kidney failure, gynecomastia (spironolactone)
  - Diuretic type effect, watch timing
  - 100 mg spironolactone often used in combo with 40 mg furosemide ratio in ascites
  - Heart Failure compelling indication
- Alpha-blockers
  - Not first line for hypertension (see BPH for medication discussion)

Hyperthyroid

Signs/Symptoms/Diagnosis/Complications
- A common type of hyperthyroidism is Graves' disease
- Your body is "amped up"
- Anxiety
- Tremor
- Increased pulse/arrhythmias
- Weight loss
- Typically noted by a suppressed TSH (below normal TSH)
- Always warm, sensitive to heat
- Rarely see new onset hyperthyroidism in an elderly patient
- Bulging eyes – Graves Ophthalmology

Common Risk Factors
- Family history
- Females

Medications to Know
- Acute management of thyroid storm – Beta blockers
    - Obviously helps with tachycardia risk
- Methimazole
    - Typically will take a little while to work
- Propylthiouracil (PTU)
    - Generally avoid unless methimazole is not tolerable
    - Higher incidence of liver problems than methimazole
- Radioactive iodine or surgery are often utilized in the management of hyperthyroidism

Hypokalemia

Signs/Symptoms/Diagnosis/Complications
- Weakness, fatigue
- Muscle cramps
- Arrhythmias
- Usual range between 3.5-5.1

Common Risk Factors
- Medications
    - Diuretics (loops, thiazides, and thiazide like)
    - Insulin can abruptly cause potassium shift
- Alcohol abuse
- Diarrhea, vomiting

Medications to Know
- Potassium replacement
    - GI adverse effects
- Remove or reduce dose of offending medication (if possible)
- Can try to help boost mild hypokalemia with medications commonly used in CHF, diabetes, hypertension etc. (i.e. aldosterone antagonists, ACE/ARBs)

Hyponatremia

Signs/Symptoms/Diagnosis/Complications
- Central Nervous System changes
    - Fatigue
    - Confusion
    - Changes in behavior, irritability
    - Headache
    - Nausea and vomiting
    - Normal sodium usually in 135-145 range
        - <130 start to get a little more concern
    - Quick drop is typically more risky than chronic hyponatremia
- Severe hyponatremia
    - Seizures
    - Brain swelling
    - Coma

Common Risk Factors
- Syndrome of Inappropriate Antidiuretic Hormone (SIADH)
    - ADH causes water retention and resulting dilution of sodium leading to hyponatremia
- Common medications that cause hyponatremia
    - Diuretics
    - SSRI's (possibly SNRI's) via SIADH
    - Carbamazepine via SIADH
    - Chlorpropamide via SIADH
- Dehydration
    - Fluid/sodium intake is reduced
    - Severe vomiting and diarrhea
- States where the body has excessive fluid without electrolytes
    - Drinking too much water
    - Heart failure (uncontrolled)
- Age

Medications to Know
- Treating chronic hyponatremia
    - Remove offending agent
    - Correct identifiable problem
    - Clinical monitoring important (i.e. are they showing signs/symptoms)
- Sodium chloride tablets
- Demeclocycline

- Tetracycline derivative
- GI side effects
- Sun sensitivity
- Expensive

Hypothyroid

Signs/Symptoms/Diagnosis/Complications
- Can mimic some signs/symptoms of depression
    - TSH should be considered a differential diagnosis in our elderly population who are experiencing signs/symptoms of depression
- Normal lab 0.5-6 (can vary depending upon the lab)
    - Hypothyroidism typically noted by an elevated TSH
    - Subclinical hypothyroidism involves abnormal TSH (usually slightly elevated) with no to minimal clinical symptoms of hypothyroidism
- Fatigue
- Incidence can increase with age
- Constipation
- Weight gain
- Sensitivity to cold
- Thinning hair
- Slower heart rate
- Dry skin
- CNS impairment
- Classic medications that can cause or contribute hypothyroidism
    - Lithium
    - Amiodarone
- Thyroid gland produces T3 and T4
- TSH is produced by the pituitary

Common Risk Factors
- Age >60
- Preexisting autoimmune disease
- Females
- Family history
- Surgery or procedure on the thyroid gland

Medications to Know
- Levothyroxine
    - Classic binding drug interactions can reduce absorption
        - Iron, calcium, cholestyramine, and many other medications
    - Consistent administration is important (especially if TSH is fine and patient is clinically asymptomatic)
    - If you are having to increase the dose, assess

- - - Adherence
    - Potential for binding interactions and/or timing of levothyroxine
  - For patients with a G-tube, administration timing can be very important
  - Monitor TSH every 2-3 months, some will do closer to 6 weeks if really out of range and patient has significant symptoms
  - Adverse effects are signs of hyperthyroidism
    - Insomnia, anxiety, tremor, tachycardia, weight loss, increased appetite
    - Prolonged suppressed TSH can lead to osteoporosis

Influenza

Signs/Symptoms/Diagnosis/Complications
- Fever
- Aches
- Fatigue/weakness
- Cough/Wheezing
- Airborne transmission
- Complications
    - Bacterial pneumonia
    - Respiratory distress
    - Death

Common Risk Factors
- Close living arrangements
    - Long term care
    - Assisted living
    - Hospital
- High risk of complications
    - Elderly
    - Underlying respiratory disorder like COPD and asthma
    - Immunosuppressed

Medications to Know
- Oseltamivir
    - Drug of choice for prophylaxis and treatment
    - Side effects: GI, psych events possible but rare
    - Prophylaxis should target at risk patients who have been or will be exposed to other patients infected with the virus
        - Particular focus on patients who might have a high risk of negative complications
    - Dose adjustments with kidney disease
- Influenza vaccine
    - Most important preventative step
    - Annual vaccination recommended
        - Numerous strain combinations
            - Hemagglutinin and neuraminidase
    - Most will use high dose for elderly patients
        - More immune response
        - 2016-2017 ACIP still doesn't recommend high dose over standard dose
    - Injection only in elderly

- Options exist for patients with true egg allergy
- Vaccination will not treat active infection
- Usually given in the fall prior, but can vaccinate into the spring for those that haven't had it

Insomnia

Signs/Symptoms/Diagnosis/Complications
- Unable to fall asleep
- Unable to maintain sleep
- Daytime fatigue/sleepiness
- First line therapy is sleep hygiene
    - Avoid daytime napping
    - Avoid stimulants like caffeine etc. close to bedtime
    - Exercise early in the day
    - Stay on a routine schedule
    - Avoid stimulating activities close to bedtime
    - Fresh air exposure throughout the day if possible
    - Minimizing stress

Common Risk Factors
- Medications that can exacerbate/cause insomnia
    - Corticosteroids
    - Stimulants
    - Decongestants (i.e. pseudoephedrine)
    - Caffeine
- Women
- Age > 60
- Alternating shift work
- Mental health disorders

Medications to Know
- Trazodone
    - Lower doses typically used for insomnia (12.5-100 mg) especially in the elderly
    - Classically considered an antidepressant, but usually only at higher doses
    - Orthostasis is possible
    - Generally considered to be better tolerated in the elderly than "Z" drugs or anticholinergics
- "Z" Drugs (i.e. zolpidem, zaleplon etc.)
    - Very similar adverse effect profile to benzodiazepines
    - Significant increase in the risk of falls in the elderly
    - Dizziness, confusion, sedation
    - Rare sleep side effects like sleep walking/eating
    - Vivid/bad dreams possible
- Anticholinergics (diphenhydramine, doxepin)

- Many available over the counter
- Not recommended in the elderly especially on a chronic basis
- Exacerbates constipation, BPH, dry eyes, dry mouth, confusion etc.
- Melatonin
  - Available OTC
  - Considered "safe" by many patients due to it being a natural product
  - Side effects of dizziness, GI, headache, lingering sedation throughout the day
  - Not great clinical trial evidence of effectiveness, but some patients will swear by it
  - Maybe not a terrible option versus anticholinergics and Z drugs
- Benzodiazepines (see anxiety for adverse effects)
  - Shorter acting used
    - i.e. Triazolam, Temazepam
- Ramelteon
  - Still expensive at this time
  - Acts on melatonin receptors
  - Dizziness, GI side effects
- Mirtazapine
  - Often used at low doses for its sedative properties
  - A potential option to help with insomnia, weight loss, and mental health disorder like depression or possibly anxiety

Irritable Bowel Syndrome

Signs/Symptoms/Diagnosis/Complications
- Abdominal pain/cramping
- Bloated feeling
- Patients with IBS can have constipation or diarrhea (usually one is predominant however)
- Blood loss or weight loss could indicate something else is going on
- Selection of chronic medications for other disease states is very important (i.e. avoid medications that may worsen the predominant symptom)
    - If IBS with constipation is predominant, avoid or try to minimize TCA's, Opioids, Calcium channel blockers etc.
    - If IBS with diarrhea is predominant, avoid or try to minimize use of sertraline, donepezil, colchicine etc.
- Recognition and avoidance of triggers is important – possible triggers;
    - Stress
    - Various foods
    - Certain medications

Common Risk Factors
- Women
- Usual onset in younger patients <45
- Family history

Medications to Know
- Fiber with fluids for constipation
    - Typical constipation medications may be tried
        - PEG or Milk of mag
        - Stool softeners (i.e. docusate)
        - Stimulants (i.e. bisacodyl)
    - Lubiprostone approved, but expensive at this time
- Diarrhea symptom management
    - Loperamide (opioid activity, but limited to the gut at low doses)
    - Diphenoxylate/atropine
        - Controlled substance
    - Cholestyramine
        - Cholesterol medication
        - Can help bulk up stools
        - Lots of binding interactions with other medications that can reduce absorption

- o   Colestipol
    - ▪ Constipating (which is what we would use it for)
- Pain/cramping/diarrhea
    - o   May see TCA's utilized
    - o   Dicyclomine
    - o   Hyoscyamine

Malnutrition

Signs/Symptoms/Diagnosis/Complications
- Lack of adequate nutrition
- Weakness, muscle loss
- Falls
- Fractures
- Possible reduction in immune function
- Reduced healing of wounds
- Reduction in body weight

Common Risk Factors
- Dementia
- Financial/income concerns
- Social isolation
- Depression
- Alcohol abuse
- Diet changes (i.e. medical diets)
- Reduced taste/smell sensations as we age

Medications to Know
- Medications that can help stimulate appetite
    - Mirtazapine
        - See depression
    - Dronabinol
        - Not ideal to use in elderly population
        - CNS side effects (i.e. confusion, sedation)
    - Megestrol
        - Risk of edema
        - Rare reports of possible blood clots
- Medications that can suppress appetite and cause weight loss/malnutrition
    - Stimulants which are sometimes used off label for depression/rehab
        - i.e. methylphenidate
    - Acetylcholinesterase inhibitors
        - i.e. donepezil, rivastigmine
    - Digoxin toxicity

Menopause Complications

Signs/Symptoms/Diagnosis/Complications
- Menstrual cycle ends
- Loss of estrogen
- Hot flashes
- Fatigue
- Mood/depression related concerns
- Vaginal atrophy/dryness
- Night sweats
- Insomnia
- Weight gain
- Risks associated with post menopause
    - Osteoporosis
    - Cardiovascular disease
    - Incontinence
    - Sexual problems (decreased libido, vaginal dryness etc.)

Common Risk Factors
- Age 40's – 50's
    - Symptoms can linger into 60's+
- Family history of difficult menopause transition

Medications to Know
- Hormone replacement therapy
    - If patients need to use estrogen replacement
        - Minimize length of therapy if possible
        - Minimize dose if possible
    - Increase risk of
        - DVT/PE
        - Breast Cancer
        - Heart disease, stroke
- Topical estrogen
    - Beneficial for vaginal dryness
    - Less systemic risk than oral estrogen
- Medications that may be helpful for menopausal symptoms like hot flashes, mood changes
    - SNRI's
        - Venlafaxine
    - SSRI's
        - Paroxetine, fluoxetine
    - Anticonvulsants

- Gabapentin

Multiple Sclerosis

Signs/Symptoms/Diagnosis/Complications
- Muscle weakness
    - Can lead to paralysis
- Visual problems
- Problems with bladder
- Difficulty walking/coordinating movements
    - Can greatly increase risk of falling
- Dizziness
- Tremor possible
- Numbness or tingling
- Relapsing remitting disease common
    - Periods of significant symptoms followed by periods of minimal symptoms or asymptomatic
- At greater risk of depression
- Mental status changes possible

Common Risk Factors
- Typically younger age onset teens-50's
- Family history
- Women
- Epstein Barr history
- Smoking
- Northern European descent

Medications to Know
- Corticosteroids
    - Often used for MS attacks
- Beta-interferons
    - Reduces the rate of relapses
    - Injection site reaction – influenza type symptoms
        - May pretreat with acetaminophen or NSAIDs
- Glatiramer
    - Itching, irritation at injection site
- Muscle relaxants/antispasmodic medications are often used
    - Tizanidine
        - Sedation, confusion
    - Baclofen
        - Sedation, dizziness, constipation
    - Cyclobenzaprine
        - Anticholinergic activity is significant

- Sedation, confusion
- Generally not first line in the elderly

Nausea/Vomiting

Signs/Symptoms/Diagnosis/Complications
- Causes
    - Often can be caused by medications in our polypharmacy patient
        - Opioids
        - Acetylcholinesterase inhibitors
        - NSAIDs (typically more pain/irritation however)
        - Chemotherapy
        - Digoxin
    - Gastroparesis (diabetes)
    - Certain foods/diets
    - Motion sickness
    - Gastroenteritis/infection
    - GERD/Hiatal hernia
    - Post op
    - Migraines

Common Risk Factors
- Family history
- Motion sickness
- History of migraines
- Certain medications

Medications to Know
- Metoclopramide
    - Blocks dopamine so can negatively affect Parkinson's
    - Potential cause of Tardive Dyskinesia
        - Abnormal involuntary movements
        - May be unmasked by dose reduction or discontinuation (especially abrupt reductions after long term use)
- Prochlorperazine
    - Technically classified as an antipsychotic
    - Often used for nausea/vertigo
    - Dopamine blockade
- Chlorpromazine
    - Dopamine blockade
    - Used for N/V, also may see used for hiccups
- Serotonin receptor antagonist (5HT-3)
    - I.e. ondansetron

- - QT prolongation risk especially when used with other prolonging agents (i.e. amiodarone)
    - Possible increase in serotonin syndrome risk
- PPI's/H2 blockers
    - You may see these tried empirically
    - Attempt to rule out GERD or other GI condition contributing to nausea and vomiting

Neuropathy

Signs/Symptoms/Diagnosis/Complications
- Painful, Tingling, Burning,
- Feeling pin pricks or needles often in feet
- Weakness, numbness
- Often happens with diabetes
- Risk of falls if patients have trouble with feeling in their feet
- Infection in feet and possibility for amputation is a big risk
- Vitamin deficiencies like B12 can possible contribute to neuropathy

Common Risk Factors
- Diabetes
- Vitamin deficiencies
- Autoimmune diseases
- Chemo
    - Vinca alkaloids (i.e. vincristine)
    - Platinum compounds (i.e. cisplatin)
    - Taxanes (i.e. paclitaxel)
- Infections
    - Shingles
    - HIV
    - Epstein Barr

Medications to Know
- Antiseizure medications and SNRI's are usual drugs of choice
- Also important to identify and treat an underlying condition to minimize risk of progression/worsening of symptoms (i.e. vitamin deficiency, diabetes control)
- Gabapentin
    - Often has to be frequently dosed
    - Can accumulate in kidney impairment
        - Be aware of dose adjustments/reduction
    - May get less bang for your buck at high doses due to % absorption decreasing as dose increases (requires a transporter in the gut to get into systemic circulation which can become saturated)
    - Frequent dosing is a downside
    - Side effects
        - Dizziness, sedation, CNS effects (fall risk)
        - Edema
- Pregabalin

- o Very similar side effect profile to gabapentin
- o Definitely well known to contribute to weight gain/fluid retention (edema)
- o Cleared by the kidney, dose adjustments may be necessary in CKD
- o Avoids the dose dependent absorption issue that gabapentin has
- o Expensive at this time, which is one of the biggest downsides
- SNRI's
  - o Duloxetine
    - Potential first line choice in someone who has mood disorder like depression as well as pain/neuropathy
    - See depression for further breakdown
  - o Venlafaxine
    - Higher doses usually necessary for benefit for neuropathy/pain
- TCA's
  - o Challenging to use these medications for neuropathy in the elderly due to their high anticholinergic activity
  - o See Depression for further breakdown
- Capsaicin
  - o Rarely may see tried
  - o Topical formulation is nice to avoid systemic side effects
  - o Needs to be applied multiple times per day
  - o PRN use is NOT effective
    - It needs to be used on a consistent basis usually for a couple of weeks to show benefit
    - Depletes substance P over time
  - o Can be irritating to skin as it is derived from peppers
- Lidocaine patches
  - o Very useful for localized areas
  - o Remember 12 hours on/12 hours off
  - o Expensive and often regulatory/insurance issues with this limits use
  - o Can cut patches
  - o Can use multiple patches (3)
  - o Systemic side effects rare when used appropriately

Oncology Complications

Signs/Symptoms/Diagnosis/Complications
- Nausea and vomiting
- Neuropathy
- Mucositis

Common Risk Factors
- Chemotherapy Induced Nausea and Vomiting
    - Higher risk – female, age >65, history of motion sickness
    - Examples of moderate to high risk chemo
        - Platinum compounds
        - Doxorubicin/daunorubicin
        - Cyclophosphamide
- Neuropathy
    - Higher risk
        - Platinum compounds
        - Vincristine
- Mucositis
    - Causes
        - 5-FU
        - Radiation

Medications to Know
- Common agents used – Chemo induced nausea and vomiting
    - Serotonin antagonists (i.e. ondansetron)
    - Neurokinin-1 receptor antagonists (i.e. aprepitant)
    - Dexamethasone
    - Prochlorperazine
    - Metoclopramide
    - Olanzapine
- Common agents used – neuropathy
    - Gabapentin
    - SNRI
    - Pregabalin
    - TCA's
        - Generally avoid in elderly if possible
- Common prevention/treatment of mucositis
    - Ice chips
    - Peridex (chlorhexidine)
    - Biotene for dry mouth
    - Diphenhydramine, lidocaine, Maalox combinations
    - Simple analgesics for pain

- Steroids for worsening cases

Orthostasis

Signs/Symptoms/Diagnosis/Complications
- Dizziness upon rising (positional changes)
- May also feel faint, nauseated, confused, light headed, weak
- Loss of baroreceptor reflex to keep adequate blood flow to the brain
- Major risks
    - Falls
    - Inadequate blood flow to brain/heart leading to potential damage
- Common cause is medication effects
    - Antihypertensives
    - Antipsychotics
    - Levodopa/carbidopa
    - Dopamine agonists
    - Sexual dysfunction medications
- Potential medical causes
    - Parkinson's
    - Bradycardia
    - Hypoglycemia
    - Afib
    - Inadequate perfusion
        - Anemia
        - Dehydration
        - Dialysis
- Compression stockings may be a potential non-drug intervention

Common Risk Factors
- Age (loss of baroreceptor reflex)
- Medications
- Medical conditions as mentioned above
- Exposure to heat/dehydration risk
- Dialysis

Medications to Know
- Primary goal is to minimize medications that can contribute to orthostasis
- If primary goal is not effective in helping, then medications can be utilized
- Fludrocortisone
    - Mineralocorticoid activity

- - Causes fluid retention which can help raise blood pressure and reduce the risk of orthostasis
  - Many adverse effects similar to corticosteroids
- Midodrine
  - Alpha agonist
  - Clamps down on vessels to raise blood pressure and reduce the risk of orthostasis
  - Opposite of alpha blocker
    - May negatively impact urinary flow (cause BPH exacerbation)

Osteoarthritis

Signs/Symptoms/Diagnosis/Complications
- Joint pain
    - Knees, hands, hips, spine most commonly affects
    - Tenderness at joint
    - Loss/damage of cartilage over time
    - Stiff, especially in the morning or after resting for a longer period of time
    - Minimal to no swelling/inflammation/redness (more typical with Rheumatoid Arthritis)
    - If joint issues become bad enough, may require replacement (i.e. knee)
    - Narrowing of joint space on x-ray

Common Risk Factors
- Age
- Obesity
- Previous injuries
- Female
- Repetitive motions

Medications/Treatments to Know
- Remember non-drug interventions
    - Physical activity can be beneficial
    - Weight management
    - Heat and/or ice
    - Physical Therapy
- Acetaminophen
    - Usual first line for osteoarthritis
    - Usually very tolerable, even in the elderly (much more so than NSAIDs)
    - Liver toxicity only concerning at >4 grams (possibly less if patient is already at risk for liver failure, i.e. cirrhosis)
    - Patient education, monitoring of combo opioid products and use of the over-the-counters incredibly important to avoid accidental overdose
    - Acetylcysteine is antidote
- NSAIDs
    - Naproxen, ibuprofen, diclofenac, meloxicam
    - Lots of concerns with NSAIDs in our elderly population, consider a potential option following adequate trial of acetaminophen

- If necessary, use short term and/or minimize dose
- GI bleed risk (especially patients with history of GI bleed/issues, on anticoagulants or antiplatelet medications)
- Impact platelet function
  - Can increase risk surrounding bleeding with surgical procedures
- CHF exacerbation risk
- Can contribute to resistant hypertension
- Possible negative impact on kidney function (especially in combo with ACE/ARB and/or diuretics)
- Avoid very high risk GI NSAIDs for OA (i.e. indomethacin and ketorolac) if possible
- Monitoring parameters
  - Kidney function
  - CBC (anemia/bleed risk)
- Naproxen dosed less often than ibuprofen which patients may like

- Mild Opioid
  - Tramadol
  - Max of 300mg in the elderly (differs from usual 400 mg)
  - Be careful in elderly as they may have seizure disorder or condition that may predispose them to seizures
  - Serotonin activity (caution in patients who are receiving high doses or multiple other serotonergic drugs
  - Sedation, constipation, dizziness, CNS effects
  - Risk of dependence/addiction, controlled substance
- Stronger opioids
  - Oxycodone, hydrocodone, morphine, fentanyl, methadone, hydromorphone, codeine
  - Class risks
    - Constipation (for chronic use likely will require stimulants and/or stool softener like docusate)
    - Sedation
    - CNS effects like confusion
    - Respiratory depression (typically in overdose)
    - No ceiling dose
    - Tolerance
    - Dependence
    - Addiction (End of life, hospice situations, we obviously don't worry about this issue much, at least with the patient)

- *Remember that opioid conversions are an approximation and that there can be multiple factors that affect pharmacokinetics; one of the major player that can impact this is pharmacogenetics; Common approximate oral equivalents:
  - Morphine 30 mg
  - Oxycodone 20 mg
  - Hydrocodone 30 mg
  - Fentanyl 12 mcg/hour patch
- Cross taper at higher doses
      - Morphine
        - Gold standard for conversion (multiple dosage forms, i.e. oral, rectal, injectable etc.)
        - Caution in renal impairment
        - Long acting and short acting available
      - Oxycodone
        - Combo with acetaminophen option
        - Oral only
        - Long acting and short acting available
      - Hydrocodone
        - In combo with acetaminophen
        - Approximate potency equivalent to morphine
      - Fentanyl patch
        - Long onset/long offset – not appropriate for acute pain relief or as needed use
        - Can cover with a Tegaderm patch or another adhesive
        - Heat can increase rate of absorption – avoid
      - Codeine
        - 2D6 converts to morphine
        - Rapid metabolizer of 2D6 will lead to more opioid effects
        - Drugs that inhibit 2D6 will lead to less opioid effects
        - Less potent than morphine, oxycodone etc.
      - Methadone
        - Conversion from or to methadone is a huge burden
        - Highest QTC prolongation risks of any opioids
          - Careful with other QTC prolonging meds
      - Meperidine
        - Do not use in the elderly
        - Risk of CNS effects including seizure
- Topical agents can be helpful especially if only a joint or two is affected by osteoarthritis

- Menthol type product, salicylate (i.e. Bengay)
- Topical NSAID – (I.e. diclofenac gel)
- Capsaicin
- Glucosamine/Chondroitin
    - Target dose of 1500mg/day glucosamine
    - Takes time to work (weeks to months)
    - Might be worth a consideration to avoid other higher risk classes in elderly like NSAIDs and opioids

Osteomyelitis

Signs/Symptoms/Diagnosis/Complications
- Infection of the bone
    - Pain, swelling at site of infection
    - Systemic symptoms possible (i.e. fever)
- Often caused by surgery, or trauma where bone may be exposed to pathogen (joint replacement is a common cause)
- Bacteria from the blood stream can possibly cause this as well
- Length of treatment is often several weeks (4-6+)
- Osteonecrosis (death of bone tissue) is possible
- Surgical interventions may be used
    - Removal of infected bone (debridement)
    - Amputation if infection is unlikely to be healed by medication therapy and patients have inadequate blood perfusion
- If osteomyelitis is likely from a non-healthcare source, the infection may be polymicrobial
- If osteomyelitis is from a healthcare setting, drug resistant pathogens need to be considered (i.e. MRSA)

Common Risk Factors
- Uncontrolled diabetes, and inadequate healing/blood flow especially to lower parts of the body can increase the risk of osteomyelitis
- Peripheral arterial disease (PAD)
- IV Drug abusers
- Recent fracture and/or surgery involving the bones
- Immunosuppression

Medications to Know
- Rifampin
    - Common add on medication as it can help prevent biofilm and infection from recurring
    - Notorious enzyme inducer (reduces levels of medications that are metabolized by various CYP enzymes – i.e. warfarin, phenytoin)
- Clindamycin
    - Good coverage against anaerobes
    - MRSA coverage
    - Frequent administration is kind of a nuisance – usually 3-4 times per day
    - Recommended to give with a full glass of water to minimize esophageal ulceration risk

- o Topical formulation also available (acne or bacterial vaginosis)
- Vancomycin
  - o MRSA coverage
  - o If red man syndrome happens, should be able to slow infusion rate to help treat
  - o Trough concentration and kidney function are important to help guide dosing
  - o You should never see this medication taken orally (one exception is a GI infection like C. Diff) – it has poor oral absorption into the blood circulation through the GI tract'
  - o 10-20 is target trough level – higher end for more serious/life threatening infections
- Linezolid
  - o MRSA and VRE coverage
  - o MAOI activity so may need to hold or adjust antidepressants that can increase serotonin (SSRI's, TCA's etc.)
  - o Oral and IV available
  - o Expensive
  - o Rare AE's like myelosuppression (bone marrow suppression, low WBC etc.) and lactic acidosis
- Levofloxacin
  - o Commonly used to cover gram negative pathogens

Osteoporosis

Signs/Symptoms/Diagnosis/Complications
- Typically asymptomatic until fracture
- DEXA scan
- T-score -2.5 or lower
- Osteopenia T-score (-1 to -2.5)

Common risk factors
- Age (bone mass starts declining around age 30)
- Female
- Postmenopausal
- Family history
- Cigarette smoking
- Hyperthyroidism
- Corticosteroid use
- Rheumatoid arthritis

Medications to Know
- Calcium
    - Target intake 1,200 to 2,000 mg/day
    - Citrate may be better absorbed in certain situations
    - Binding interactions (quinolones, levothyroxine, tetracycline's etc.)
    - Found in many common OTC antacids (calcium carbonate)
    - Constipating
- Vitamin D
    - Replacement 50,000 units weekly for 8-12 weeks
    - Usual maintenance 1,000-2,000 units per day
    - Target level >30-35, some may argue higher
- Bisphosphonates
    - Esophageal concerns with oral
    - Educate patient about administration procedure (upright for 30-60 minutes, full glass of plain water, with no other meds etc.)
    - Examples; risedronate, alendronate, ibandronate
    - Zoledronic Acid (once yearly) – concerns with acute renal failure especially patients CrCl less than 35 mls/min
- Denosumab
    - 2 times per year injection
    - Targets RANKL
    - Seems to be growing in popularity

- - - o SE's – low calcium, muscle pain, injection pain, weakness
- SERM
    - o Example: raloxifene
    - o Risk of DVT, stroke, and hot flashes
    - o Makes sense especially in patients who have indication for breast cancer
- Parathyroid
    - o Teriparatide
    - o Anabolic (works on building bone – osteoblasts)
    - o Lab monitoring parathyroid hormone (PTH) and calcium/vitamin D
    - o ONLY use for 2 years
- Calcitonin
    - o Nasal spray (also subQ, but rarely ever used)
    - o Can have benefit for compression fracture pain
- Estrogen Therapy
    - o Beneficial for osteoporosis, but avoid due to risks of cancer, clots etc.
    - o Possible use in patients who can't/won't come off estrogen for postmenopausal symptoms

Pancreatitis

Signs/Symptoms/Diagnosis/Complications
- Upper quadrant abdominal pain
- Pain can radiate to different areas
- Nausea/vomiting
- Tenderness when touching or possibly with movement
- Pain likely worse following eating

Common Risk Factors
- Alcohol use
- Gallstone history
- Elevated triglycerides (target triglycerides at 500 or higher)
- Lots of meds could contribute, but all are fairly rare
    - Timing will likely be an important factor to look at

Medications to Know
- Fibrates
    - i.e. fenofibrate, gemfibrozil
    - GI Side effects
    - Gemfibrozil tends to have a higher risk of rhabdomyolysis than fenofibrate
        - Use fenofibrate if possible when patient is already receiving a statin
- Niacin
    - Can possibly increase HDL as well as lower TG's
    - Best to avoid if possible in patients with gout as can raise uric acid
    - Flushing side effect
        - Can be helped with aspirin, but likely want to avoid higher doses of aspirin in our high risk elderly population
- Fish Oil
    - GI upset
    - Fishy taste
        - Can help to put in fridge
    - Large pills to swallow can be challenging for patients
    - Possible impact on platelet function (theoretical bleed risk)

Parkinson's Disorder

Signs/Symptoms/Diagnosis/Complications
- Shortage of dopamine in the brain
- "TRAP"
    o Tremor at rest
    o Rigidity or "stiffness" in movement
    o Akinesia (inability to move when desired)
    o Postural changes/instability
- Patients with Parkinson's can have a high rate of falls
- Dopamine agonists can worsen Parkinson's; classic examples
    o Antipsychotics
    o Metoclopramide
- Often patients will have swallowing difficulties as time goes on
    o Aspiration pneumonia risk
- Other complications
    o Constipation
    o Loss of bladder control/incontinence
    o Depression
    o Lewy Body dementia
    o Behavioral changes
    o Orthostasis

Common Risk Factors
- Genetics
- Males
- Head trauma
- Age

Medications to Know
- Sinemet (Carbidopa/levodopa) – dopamine replacement
    o Gold standard for treatment
    o Does not reverse Parkinson's, simply treats the symptoms
    o Adverse effects
        ▪ GI (Nausea/vomiting)
        ▪ Hallucinations – due to excessive dopamine
        ▪ Orthostasis
        ▪ Dyskinesia (involuntary movements)
    o Frequent dosing – controlled release can help reduce pill burden
    o Taking with significant protein in the diet can affect absorption
- Dopamine agonists

- o Option in mild to moderate Parkinson's disorder
- o See Restless leg for further breakdown
- Catechol-O-methyltransferase inhibitors
  - o Entacapone, tolcapone
  - o Help prevent breakdown of levodopa
  - o May have to reduce levodopa (Sinemet) dosing when initiating or at least monitor for signs of Sinemet toxicity
  - o Not effective if given alone (i.e. not with levodopa
  - o Tolcapone – rarely used, hepatotoxicity risk
  - o Adverse effects: look out for increased Sinemet concentrations (so adverse effects will look like Sinemet toxicity)
- MAOI's
  - o Selegiline, rasagiline
  - o Prevent the breakdown of dopamine
  - o Selectively target MAO – type B
    - Tyramine/food interaction less likely than MAOI's used for depression
- Anticholinergics
  - o Rarely used due to adverse effect profile in elderly
- Amantadine
  - o May see used to help with levodopa side effect of dyskinesia
  - o Adverse effects
    - Edema
    - Purple spots on the skin
    - Hallucinations

Peptic Ulcer Disease

Signs/Symptoms/Diagnosis/Complications
- Stomach pain
- Bleeding (black tarry stools)
- Often associated with heartburn
- Occult blood positive
- Can cause anemia
- Gastric ulcer – stomach
- Duodenal in the duodenum
- H. pylori and NSAIDs are the two most common causes
    - Breath test for H pylori testing

Common Risk Factors
- NSAID use
- Corticosteroid use
- Smoking
- Alcohol use

Medications to Know
- OAC or MOC are two common treatments of H. pylori
    - Omeprazole, amoxicillin, clarithromycin
    - Or metronidazole, omeprazole, clarithromycin
    - Typically 14 day course of treatment
    - May also see tetracycline and/or bismuth used
- PPI's
    - See GERD
- Metronidazole
    - Avoid alcohol use
    - Interaction via 2C9 (warfarin is the big one)
    - GI side effects most common
    - Can cause abnormal taste
- Clarithromycin
    - Macrolide
    - 3A4 inhibition – lots of drug interactions
    - GI side effects
    - QTc prolongation risk
- Amoxicillin
    - See pneumonia
- Bismuth subsalicylate
    - Neurotoxicity rare, but possible with unsupervised very high doses

- - Salicylate component can theoretically increase bleeding risk
  - Grey/black discoloration of the stool
- Avoidance of NSAIDs, corticosteroids
  - If necessary, use prophylaxis with PPI or H2 blocker if PPI intolerable

Peripheral Artery Disease

Signs/Symptoms/Diagnosis/Complications
- Lack of blood flow to legs, extremities
- Causes claudication
    - Pain when walking as demand for blood flow/oxygen increases
- Symptoms will get worse the further the patient tries to walk
- Sharp, cramping, sometimes numbness type pain usually relieved by resting for a period of time
    - Calf muscle often affected
- Atherosclerosis, narrowing of the arteries is the usual cause
- May see wounds that won't heal (inadequate blood flow)
- Risk of amputation
- Pedal pulse absent or very weak

Common Risk Factors
- Smoking
- Diabetes
- Obesity
- High cholesterol
- High blood pressure

Medications to Know
- Statins
- Treat hypertension
- Manage diabetes
- Antiplatelet therapy (aspirin or clopidogrel if aspirin contraindication)
- First line is the above measures, may see clinicians try these if no response
- Cilostazol
    - Mechanism not completely understood
        - Antiplatelet activity
        - Opens up vessels
    - Administer on empty stomach
    - GI side effects, headache
- Pentoxifylline
    - Give with food
    - Well tolerated overall
    - GI side effects if anything

Physiological and Lifestyle Changes in the Elderly

Heart and Vessels
- Atherosclerosis
    - Increased MI/Stroke risk
- Reduced cardiac output
- Increased stiffness of vessels
    - Hypertension
- Reduced baroreceptor reflex
    - Orthostasis risk

Body Composition
- Reduced muscle mass
    - Can cause lower serum creatinine as muscle mass declines
    - Reduced physical activity/conditioning
- Bone loss (osteoporosis)
- Increase in fat
    - Can alter pharmacokinetics of lipophilic drugs
- Often reduced water
    - Dehydration risk

Skin
- Dryness
- Cracking
- Infection risk
- Skin thinning

Immune System
- Reduced function
- Increased susceptibility to infection
- Opportunistic pathogens possible

GI Tract
- Slowed GI tract
- Reduced absorption of some elements/vitamins
    - Iron - Reduced acidity
    - B12 – Reduced intrinsic factor
- Oral/dental care can impact oral intake

Senses
- Visual impairments (i.e. glaucoma, macular degeneration)
    - Quality of life concerns
        - Driving, reading etc.
- Reduced taste/smell

- Can contribute to weight loss
- Hearing impairments
    - Can greatly impact patient education, risk for errors and patient mistakes
- Touch
    - Neuropathy and other conditions can impact this sensation

Kidney Function
- Reduced kidney function
    - Accumulation of drugs that are eliminated by the kidney
- Reduced capacity to produce erythropoietin

Reflexes
- Reduced reflexes can increase risk of balance problems/falls

Blood composition
- Reduced albumin which can increase free fraction of highly protein bound drugs
- Anemia of chronic disease
- Reduced erythropoietin production (especially in CKD)
- Infection risk, reduced white blood cell production

Respiratory
- Reduced lung capacity/function
- Reduced oxygen saturations

Reduced hormone production
- Estrogen
- Testosterone
- Hypothyroid concerns
    - Reduced metabolism can contribute to weight gain

Social Concerns
- Loneliness
- Loss of independence
- Impacts on self-esteem/self-worth
- Suicide risk
- Mood/anxiety issues
- Caregiver burnout
- Fear of institutionalization
- Fear of moving

Financial
- Costs of care
    - Long term care

- - Assisted living
  - Hospitalization
  - Home care
- Lack of income or fixed incomes
- Risk of falling for financial scams
- Friends/family taking advantage of them
  - Elder abuse – intentional, knowledge of, or negligent act by caregiver or other individual toward a vulnerable adult

Pneumonia

Signs/Symptoms/Diagnosis/Complications
- Shortness of breath
- Chest discomfort/pain
- Possible fever (less common in the elderly)
- Green/yellow sputum
- Fatigue
- GI upset
- Strep pneumoniae is most common pathogen
- Mycoplasma often termed "walking pneumonia"
- Aspiration pneumonia common in the elderly due to reduced capacity of the swallowing/GI system (contents more likely to be inhaled into the lung)

Common Risk Factors
- Smoking
- COPD
- Asthma
- Immunocompromised
- Hospitalized
- Risk factors that may require hospitalization
    - Age >65
    - Tachypnea (>30 breaths per minute)
    - Hypotension (<90/60)
    - Confusion
    - Elevated BUN

Medications to Know
- It is incredibly important to understand resistance patterns throughout your area as this may be one of the determining factors for antibiotic selection
- Macrolides (often used in combo with beta-lactam or sometimes cephalosporin)
    - Uncomplicated, low risk of hospitalization, you may see azithromycin used alone
    - May run into Strep pneumo resistance in some areas
    - Considered more active versus atypical pathogens compared to beta-lactams
    - GI adverse effects
    - Administration is easy due to long half-life (once daily dosing)
    - Possible QTC prolongation risk

- Beta-lactam (amoxicillin, amoxicillin/clavulanate)
    - GI side effects are most common
        - Diarrhea especially
    - Sometimes used in combo with azithromycin to help Strep pneumo coverage for community acquired pneumonia
- Cephalosporins (i.e. ceftriaxone)
    - Injection necessary (ceftriaxone)
    - Broader spectrum coverage than amoxicillin
    - More likely to be used as risk stratification for hospitalization gets higher
- Tetracycline derivatives (i.e. doxycycline)
    - Often used if penicillin allergy
    - Nice oral option for outpatient therapy
    - Photosensitivity
    - Binding interaction with metal cations (i.e. iron etc.)
    - Twice daily dosing
    - Option if MRSA suspected or confirmed
- Respiratory fluoroquinolones (i.e. levofloxacin, moxifloxacin)
    - Generally considered a "bigger gun", reserved for more resistant bugs and patients at higher risk for hospitalization/complication
        - FDA warnings on avoiding use for less serious infections like sinusitis, uncomplicated UTI's, bronchitis
    - QTC prolongation risk
    - Spontaneous tendon rupture
    - Binding interactions (i.e. iron, calcium etc.)
- Hospital or ventilator associated
    - Broader spectrum antibiotics
        - Pip/tazo
        - Cefepime
        - Respiratory fluoroquinolone
        - Penems (imipenem, meropenem)
    - MRSA suspected
        - Vancomycin
        - Linezolid
        - Avoid daptomycin
- Pneumococcal vaccination very important – see Vaccines section

Restless Legs

Signs/Symptoms/Diagnosis/Complications
- Creeping, painful, uncomfortable feeling in the legs
- Often worse when patients are not moving
    - Sleeping or at rest
- More often in middle aged or older patients
- Will sometimes see accompanied with the following conditions
    - Parkinson's
    - Iron deficiency (assess ferritin, iron stores)
    - Neuropathy
- No medical test for diagnosis, however, it would be appropriate to rule out iron deficiency

Common Risk Factors
- Iron deficiency
- Parkinson's
- Kidney Disease
- Neuropathy

Medications to Know
- Dopamine agonists; pramipexole, ropinirole
    - Often will be dosed at night as that's when many patients will have symptoms, but can be dosed during the day as well
    - Adverse effects
        - Sedation
        - Orthostasis
        - Possible psych related concerns (agonist at dopamine, remember that schizophrenia is characterized by too much dopamine)
        - Edema
        - Rare, reports of obsessive type behaviors (i.e. gambling)
- Gabapentin, pregabalin
    - See Neuropathy
- Sinemet (levodopa/carbidopa)
    - If you see this dose once daily (typically at night), you can likely suspect that it is being used for RLS versus multiple times throughout the day which is often necessary in Parkinson's disorder
    - May be used as needed
    - See Parkinson's for bigger breakdown

- Iron supplementation if deficiency
    - Assess ferritin level

Rheumatoid Arthritis

Signs/Symptoms/Diagnosis/Complications
- Autoimmune disorder
    - Osteoarthritis is more of an overuse, chronic issue over time
- Treatment involves use of agents that reduce inflammation and suppresses immune system
- Painful, swollen, redness, warmth in joints
- May see systemic effects like fever and fatigue
- Irreversible damage of the 'lining' of the joints can occur
- Deformities in the joints (slanted hands)
- PIP joints often affected
- Hands, wrists impacted – can limit/impair daily routine tasks
- Females more likely to be diagnosed with RA than males
- Early diagnosis, early intervention initiation of DMARD important
- Increases risk for osteoporosis
- Infection risk (especially when many of the medications suppress immune function)
- Patients with RA may have elevated C-reactive protein (CRP) as well as elevated Erythrocyte Sedimentation Rate (ESR)

Common Risk Factors
- Middle age for diagnosis – 40-60 y/o
- Smoking
- Obesity
- Family history
- Female

Medications to Know
- DMARD
    - DMARDs delay the progression and worsening of the disease
        - Examples: Methotrexate, hydroxychloroquine, sulfasalazine, azathioprine
        - Monitor CBC, LFT
        - Watch immunosuppression risk (WBC)
        - DMARDs do not work quickly…takes weeks to months
    - Methotrexate
        - Once weekly dosing
        - Folic acid supplementation
        - Liver toxicity risk
        - Injection available if difficulty with oral

- Sulfasalazine
    - GI side effects most common
    - Can impair folic acid absorption
    - Twice daily dosing
- Hydroxychloroquine
    - Routine eye exams necessary
    - LFT's
- Azathioprine
    - See Crohn's

- Corticosteroids
    - Example: Prednisone, methylprednisolone
    - Usual use is to treat an acute flare of RA
    - Reduces inflammation
    - Minimize length of therapy if at all possible
    - Immune suppression risk
    - Exacerbates diabetes – causes hyperglycemia
    - Can cause GI upset, increase ulcer risk
    - Insomnia, anxiety
    - HPA suppression risk
    - Osteoporosis risk if used longer term
    - Heart failure risk
    - Increase hypertension
    - Possible increase risk of elevated intraocular pressure (monitor in patients on longer term use) – glaucoma
- NSAIDs
    - Usually intended for short term relief of inflammation in RA flares
    - See osteoarthritis for medication breakdown

Schizophrenia

Signs/Symptoms/Diagnosis/Complications
- "Positive symptoms"
    - Hallucinations
    - Delusions
    - Altered sense of reality
    - Psychosis
- Negative symptoms
    - Socially withdrawn
    - Flat affect
    - Inability to function normally in life
- Onset in younger adults
- Suicide/drug abuse/other mental health concerns often an issue
- Difficult for patients to remain adherent to drug therapy

Common Risk Factors
- Family history
- Taking psychoactive drugs younger in life

Medications to Know
- Antipsychotic selection based on multiple factors
    - Adverse effect profile
    - Convenience
    - Dosage forms
    - Adherence
- Rarely are first generation antipsychotics (i.e. haloperidol) used due to very high rates of extra pyramidal side effects
- Atypical examples (second generation); clozapine, risperidone, aripiprazole, quetiapine, ziprasidone, olanzapine
- Risperidone, paliperidone has highest risk of elevated prolactin levels
- Aripiprazole has lowest risk of elevating prolactin levels
- Olanzapine, clozapine have highest risk of metabolic syndrome
    - Likely will avoid in overweight, diabetes, high cardiac risk
- Quetiapine has lowest risk of extrapyramidal effects (due to least potent dopamine blockade)
    - May be advantageous in patients who experience EPS with other agents, Parkinson's or other movement disorders
- Clozapine, quetiapine considered more sedating
- Aripiprazole, Ziprasidone have lowest risk for metabolic syndrome
- Clozapine last line due to agranulocytosis risk, frequent WBC, ANC lab monitoring

- Periodically monitor for metabolic syndrome in patients on antipsychotics (lipids, A1C etc.)
- Long acting injectables are an option for many of the antipsychotics;
    - Make sure oral test doses are done
- QTC prolongation risk – possibly highest with ziprasidone
- Aripiprazole often used for antidepressant augmentation
- To help with movement adverse effects (EPS) and also possibly with drooling, you may see anticholinergics used; i.e. benztropine, trihexyphenidyl or diphenhydramine

Seizures

Signs/Symptoms/Diagnosis/Complications
- Absence (petit mal) – Loss of consciousness for a brief period of time
- Atonic (drop attacks) – loss of muscle tone
- Tonic-clonic (grand mal); rigidity and jerking movements
- Tonic – muscle rigidity
- Clonic – jerking movements that are repetitive
- Myoclonic – sporadic jerking

Common Risk Factors
- Traumatic Brain Injury
- Illicit drug use
- Abrupt electrolyte changes
- Older Age
- Family history
- Significant alcohol use

Medications to Know
- Phenytoin
    - Memorable Side Effects: GI, CNS changes, ataxia, vitamin D deficiency, liver function changes (rare)
    - Be on the lookout for drug interactions (a few examples: fluconazole, amiodarone, alcohol, cimetidine, fluvoxamine, etc.) – if new meds are started, I would recommend looking up potential interactions
    - Narrow therapeutic window drug - Very sensitive to changes in dose (small increase may lead to toxicity)
        - Michaelis-Menten kinetics
    - Usual phenytoin total level is from 10-20 (can be misleading if patient has low albumin), obtaining a free level is considered best, but not possible by all laboratories (target free level is generally 1-2)
    - Toxicity similar to alcohol toxicity in many ways…ataxia (difficulty walking), confusion, GI side effects like nausea, slurred speech, etc.
    - Can induce vitamin D metabolism leading to deficiency
- Levetiracetam
    - Less drug interactions
    - Levels typically not done
        - Possibly checked to assure adherence
    - CNS side effects (sedation etc.)

- - Watch accumulation with poor kidney function
  - Titrate dose based upon seizures/signs of adverse effects
- Lamotrigine
  - See Bipolar Disorder
- Phenobarbital
  - Enzyme inducer
    - Reduces concentrations of many other drugs
  - Seldom used
  - 10-40 "normal drug level"
  - CNS signs/symptoms of toxicity
    - Falls, confusion, sedation
- Valproic Acid
  - See Bipolar Disorder
- Carbamazepine
  - See Bipolar Disorder
- Topiramate
  - See headaches
- Felbamate
  - Seldom used due to hepatotoxicity

Sexual Dysfunction

Signs/Symptoms/Diagnosis/Complications
- Reduced libido/desire
- Trouble getting an erection
- Issues with keeping an erection
- Psych issues can play a role
    - Stress
    - Depression
    - Anxiety
- Classic Drug Induced Causes
    - BP meds (diuretics, beta-blockers, clonidine)
    - Psych (TCA's, SSRI's, Benzo's)
    - Drugs with significant anticholinergic activity (diphenhydramine etc.)
    - H2 blockers – especially cimetidine
    - 5-alpha reductase inhibitors (i.e. finasteride)

Common Risk Factors
- Hypertension
- Diabetes
- Hyperlipidemia
- Hormone imbalances
- Prostate surgery
- Parkinson's

Medications to Know
- PDE-5 Inhibitors (i.e. sildenafil, vardenafil)
    - Nitrate interaction
    - Drop in blood pressure, orthostasis risk
    - Changes in vision color (rare)
- Change or minimize doses of medications that may be contributing to erectile dysfunction
- Examples:
    - Hypertension
        - Use ACE/ARBs or CCB like amlodipine
    - Depression
        - Use Mirtazapine or bupropion

Shingles

Signs/Symptoms/Diagnosis/Complications
- Caused by Varicella Zoster Virus (VZV)
- Same viral infection that causes chicken pox - reactivation
- Pain, burning, red rash, numbness, tingling – "nerve pain"
- Fluid filled blisters can form – fluid can transmit disease to anyone not vaccinated or who hasn't had the virus before
- Not very common, but can involve the eye and rarely lead to eye damage/blindness
- Postherpetic neuralgia
    - Pain syndrome that remains following resolution of the shingles flare
    - Neuropathic type pain

Common Risk Factors
- Age 50+ (highest incidence in the 60 y/o range)
- Immunosuppression
    - HIV/AIDS
    - Chemo
    - Transplant drugs

Medications to Know
- Valacyclovir, acyclovir
    - If going to use antiviral therapy, the sooner the better
    - Best within three days of initial onset
    - Acyclovir has to be dosed very frequently
    - Valacyclovir can be dosed less frequently which is an obvious advantage over acyclovir
    - GI side effects
    - Rarely liver issues can exist (especially if longer term therapy or other liver risk factors)
    - Can accumulate in CKD
        - Rarely neurotoxicity possible
        - Full glass of water is recommended with administration
- Symptomatic treatment of pain (similarities to neuropathy)
    - Gabapentin, pregabalin
    - TCA's
    - Topicals
        - Capsaicin
        - Lidocaine

- - SNRI's
  - Simple analgesics
  - Opioids
- Vaccination
  - "Zostavax"
  - Very important to prevent/minimize complications with shingles
  - Indicated at age 50+
  - Usually best given at around age 60 when highest incidence starts
  - Live vaccine
  - Storage requirements (freezer)
  - One time dose
  - Expensive
  - Insurance coverage may be a barrier for some patients

Skin and Soft Tissue Infection

Signs/Symptoms/Diagnosis/Complications
- Inflamed, red, warm to the touch area(s) on the skin
- Blistering, pain also possible
- Risk of seeding the blood stream causing systemic infection
- Infection will often start in an area that has had an opening (i.e. wound, surgical opening etc.)
- Leg(s) is usually the most common site, but infection can happen anywhere
- Most common causes; gram positives
    - Streptococcus
    - Staphylococcus

Common Risk Factors
- IV Drug abuse
- Obesity
- Damage/injury
- Preexisting skin conditions that may allow for a point of entry (eczema, chicken pox, or other condition that may lead to bleeding/cracks in the skin)
- Immunosuppressed

Medications to Know
- Outpatient Non-MRSA (MSSA) likely suspected (simple beta-lactam or cephalosporin)
    - Cephalexin
    - Dicloxacillin
- Outpatient MRSA suspected
    - Bactrim
    - Doxycycline
    - Clindamycin
- May use combinations if response not adequate which would include a beta-lactam with a MRSA oral agent (i.e. Bactrim, Doxy, Clinda)
- Inpatient options
    - Cefazolin, clindamycin, beta-lactam for simple infections
    - Vancomycin, linezolid, daptomycin potential options for MRSA
    - If pseudomonas present, add pip/tazo, imipenem, meropenem, cefepime, or ceftazidime as options

Smoking Cessation

Signs/Symptoms/Diagnosis/Complications
- Nicotine addiction
- Major risks associated with smoking
    - COPD
    - Lung cancer
    - Cardiovascular complications

Medications to Know
- Medication selection; nicotine replacement products, varenicline, and bupropion are both considered first line – either choice acceptable based on patient preference etc.
- Second line option – nortriptyline or clonidine
- Nicotine replacement products
    - Patches
    - Gum
    - Inhaler
    - Lozenge
    - Nasal Spray
    - *Vaping is not considered a nicotine replacement product (medical treatment) as there is limited long term evidence about safety; unclear if same long term risks as smoking or not at this time
- Varenicline
    - Partial nicotine agonist
    - Patients can still smoke while using this medication for the first week
    - Notorious for vivid dreams
    - Possible risk of psychiatric events, warning on risk of suicide
    - Insomnia
- Bupropion
    - See depression
- Clonidine
    - See hypertension
- Nortriptyline
    - See depression

Stroke/TIA

Signs/Symptoms/Diagnosis/Complications
- One sided drooping; can involve
    - Face, limbs
- Severe headache of unknown origin
- Slurred or incoherent speech
- Confusion
- Balance issues, dizziness, fall
- Trans Ischemic Attack
    - Temporary blockage that typically results in no residual symptoms following the episode
- Ischemic stroke
    - Most common type of stroke
    - Blood supply is blocked off to a certain area of the brain
    - Clot can be formed in/near the heart and sent through bigger vessels to the small brain vessels and get lodged
        - AKA - Thromboembolic stroke, common with atrial fibrillation
    - Atherosclerosis and a clot forming in the brain can also happen
        - Typically different pharmacotherapy is used for this compared to an embolic stroke originating in the heart
- Hemorrhagic stroke
    - Uncontrolled hypertension can significantly increase the risk
    - Loss of blood flow and adequate perfusion due to blood loss outside the vessels
    - Often complicated or caused by anticoagulants/antiplatelet medications
    - Anatomical abnormalities like an aneurysm can be a cause of this type of stroke

Common Risk Factors
- Diabetes
- Hypertension
- Heart Disease
- TIA's
- Age
- African, Indian descent
- Smoking
- Obesity
- High cholesterol

Medications to Know
- Stroke due to atrial fibrillation
    - Warfarin – see DVT
    - Apixaban – see DVT
    - Rivaroxaban – see DVT
    - Dabigatran – see DVT
- Stroke due to atherosclerosis in the brain blood vessels
    - Aspirin/dipyridamole
        - Twice daily dosing
        - Significant cost expense compared to clopidogrel
        - Extended release formulation
    - Clopidogrel
        - Used in place of aspirin/dipyridamole as a cheaper option as well as a once daily option
        - See Acute Coronary Syndrome
    - Aspirin alone
        - Alternative if clopidogrel and/or aspirin/dipyridamole ER not an option

Type 2 Diabetes

Signs/Symptoms/Diagnosis/Complications
- Polyuria
- Polydipsia
- Fatigue
- Polyphagia
- Fruity smelling urine (ketones)
- *Symptoms likely more common in type 1 diabetes, often geriatric patients will present with complications
- Complications
    - Nephropathy
    - Retinopathy
    - Neuropathy
    - Slow healing of wounds
    - Amputation risk
    - Increased cardiovascular risks

Common Risk Factors
- Obesity
- African descent
- Sedentary
- Insulin resistance
- HTN and Dyslipidemia
- History of gestational diabetes
- Common drugs that exacerbate diabetes
    - Corticosteroids
    - Antipsychotics
    - Thiazides
- Drugs that can affect diabetes
    - Beta-blockers, blunt signs of hypoglycemia

Medications/Management
- Typical treatment workflow with no relative contraindications
    - Metformin is first line
    - Then, add on Sulfonylurea, DPP-4, or possibly TZD
    - Generally 2 or 3 oral medications are used prior to using insulin especially if patient doesn't want to do injections, but starting insulin is a potential first line option in patients who present with very high blood sugars A1C>9
    - Can go to insulin sooner if very high blood sugars

- Tight control can prevent or delay progression of microvascular complications
- Hypoglycemia becomes more of a concern than tight management as patients age, get closer to end of life
- Remember cardiovascular risk factors and use of statins, antihypertensives, and aspirin
- May want to be less aggressive in starting doses and titrating these medications in the elderly
- Brittle or labile are often terms to describe patients who experience massive fluctuations in blood sugars – extremely difficult to manage
- Glucagon is to be used in the event of hypoglycemia with change in consciousness
    - Do not try to give oral glucose to a patient who may be unable to swallow – risk of aspiration
- In alert patients experiencing hypoglycemia symptoms, oral intake of sugar is first line treatment
- Blood sugar checks can often be reduced in our stable geriatric patients to improve quality of life
- In elderly patients with A1C's less than 6.0, keep a very close eye on symptoms of hypoglycemia and also their blood sugar readings
- A1C goals of <7.5 to 8.0 may be very reasonable in frail elderly population with limited life expectancy
- Hypoglycemia may be overlooked or misdiagnosed with vague symptoms reported, weakness, fatigue, confusion, falls, lethargy etc.

- Metformin
    - Very inexpensive
    - N/V/D most common
    - B12 deficiency possible, we should monitor for this periodically and especially if patients are displaying possible signs/symptoms or are on other meds (i.e. PPI's) that could potentially contribute
    - lactic acidosis (very rare, more common in patients with poor kidney function)
    - Doesn't stimulate production of insulin which is why it is not likely to cause hypoglycemia when used alone
    - Metformin is the first line medication for type 2 diabetes
    - Contraindicated with GFR less than 30 mls/min
        - In patient with GFR 30-45, it is often a challenging decision whether to use metformin or not; important to

- assess other issues with alternative diabetes medications (i.e. hypoglycemia risk with sulfonylureas, cost with DDP's, etc.)
  - Administration with a meal is recommended and can really help minimize GI upset
  - Metformin tends to not cause weight gain compared to other diabetes medications which is nice considering that many of our type 2 diabetes patients are overweight
  - Start low and go slow on the dosing due to GI side effects
- Sulfonylureas
  - Glipizide, Glyburide, Glimepiride
  - Inexpensive
  - Stimulate insulin release, so hypoglycemia is a major concern in our elderly population
  - Weight gain can be problematic in our likely already overweight diabetes population
  - Elderly can be especially at risk for hypoglycemia (chlorpropamide on Beer's list)
  - Chlorpropamide can cause SIADH (rarely used due to this and Beer's list designation)
  - Glipizide generally preferred in elderly
- DPP-4 Inhibitors
  - Sitagliptin, saxagliptin
  - Prolongs incretin effects amongst many actions
  - Incretin is responsible for promoting fullness, weight neutral to weight loss is common with these agents – nice advantage
  - Expensive
  - Sitagliptin most commonly used – be aware of dose adjustments in CKD
  - More data coming out on risks with heart failure (not as concerning as pioglitazone at this point)
  - Rare pancreatitis causes
  - Not likely to cause hypoglycemia like sulfonylureas unless used with SU's or insulin
- GLP-1 Inhibitors
  - Liraglutide, exenatide
  - N/V is the major adverse effect
  - Promotes fullness, weight loss can be a beneficial effect
  - Typically better reduction than most oral diabetes medications
  - Injection is a downside
  - Cost can be an issue for many patients
  - Rare concern with thyroid cancer

- SGLT-2 Inhibitors
    - Empagliflozin, canagliflozin
    - Caution on patient with urinary infection history (drugs increase sugar to the urine which can be food for bug)
    - Monitor K+; hyperkalemia risk especially in patients on ACE, ARB, etc.
    - Risk of ketoacidosis
    - Hypoglycemia risk not as bad as sulfonylureas
    - Caution on bone fracture risk
    - Hypotension, volume depletion risk, dehydration
- Alpha-glucosidase inhibitors
    - Acarbose, miglitol
    - Prevent breakdown of complex sugars in the gut
    - Leads to lots of GI side effects
    - GI SE's and frequent dosing make these medications seldom used
    - If patient has hypoglycemic episode, you MUST use simple sugars (i.e. glucose tablets) to treat it as complex sugars may not be broken down due to the drugs mechanism of action
    - Hypoglycemia risk typically not an issue if used alone
- TZD's
    - Pioglitazone
    - Weight gain, edema risk
    - Avoid in heart failure
    - Once daily dosing is nice
    - Hypoglycemia rare when used alone
- Glinides
    - Repaglinide
    - Stimulates insulin release
    - Hypoglycemia
    - Weight gain risk
    - Needs to be dose with meals
    - Frequent dosing can be a downside
- Long acting insulin
    - Glargine, detemir
    - Provides basal insulin throughout the day
    - Fasting blood sugars should be your focus
        - If patient is already having fasting hypoglycemia (i.e. early morning) increasing or adding long acting will bring that number down further
        - Great to use if blood sugars are consistently elevated all throughout the day

- - Rarely you may see higher doses split up to twice daily try to "even out" the dosing especially if having troubles with variable blood sugars (less volume injected, and hopefully less "peak" effect)
  - Weight gain
- Rapid acting
  - Give with meals or just prior
  - Useful in preventing/bringing down post-prandial blood sugars (those big spikes following meals)
  - Can be used just once or twice daily in Type 2
  - Sliding scale insulin
    - Treating "the number"
    - Giving insulin based upon the blood sugar at a given point in time
    - Reactive mentality, so sliding scale is recommended to be avoided if possible
    - Rare instances where it might be acceptable at least for short term time frames (i.e. patients who are sick, not eating well, hospitalized, brittle etc.)
- Intermediate Acting Insulin
  - Rarely used due to use of long acting
  - Likely scenario you will see; last line option, or patients who have been stable on their dosing for a long time and have no desire to switch what is working
- Short acting
  - Regular insulin
  - Typically given before the meal
  - Can be a challenge in cognitively impaired elderly patients who may not remember to eat or decide not to eat following dose of insulin

Ulcerative Colitis

Signs/Symptoms/Diagnosis/Complications
- Inflammation in the area of the colon
    - Crohn's can be in the small intestine
- Diarrhea, cramping, pain
- Rectal bleeding
- Fatigue
- Fever
- Feel the need to defecate, but can't
- Increases osteoporosis risk
- Increased risk of colon cancer

Common Risk Factors
- Typically begins in earlier ages (20's-30's)
- Whites, Jewish descent
- Family history

Medications to Know
- Mesalamine
    - Enema form can be helpful as typically only the colon is affective with Ulcerative Colitis versus Crohn's disease
    - Patients may not like enema form obviously
- Sulfasalazine
- Corticosteroids
    - Reserved for moderate to severe ulcerative colitis
- Azathioprine
- Biologics
    - Infliximab, adalimumab
- Symptom management
    - Psyllium – bulk up stool, try to reduce diarrhea
    - Loperamide – antidiarrheal
        - Be very cautious with antidiarrheal agents as they can potentially cause toxic megacolon
    - Acetaminophen – pain (remember to avoid NSAIDs)
    - Chronic bleeding (assess need for iron and B12)
- Surgery is curative for ulcerative colitis, but patients will likely have to have an ostomy bag
    - Big differentiator with Crohn's disease

Urinary Incontinence

Signs/Symptoms/Diagnosis/Complications
- Stress Incontinence
    - Caused by physical exertion (i.e. cough, rapid movement, sneeze)
    - Kegel exercises often used to help with stress incontinence
- Urge or Overactive bladder (OAB)
    - Frequently feeling like you have to go to the bathroom
- Overflow
    - Caused by a blockage of some sort
    - BPH is a very common cause of overflow incontinence (See BPH)
    - Dribbling, frequency can occur
- Functional
    - Patient who cannot physical or mentally use or get to the bathroom
    - Dementia, physical deconditioning
- Diuretics can often worsen symptoms of incontinence by increasing the volume in the bladder and increase the frequency of trips to the bathroom

Common Risk Factors
- Stress
    - Obesity
    - Childbirth (can weaken pelvic muscles)
    - Post-menopausal
    - Female
- Urge or OAB
    - MS or Parkinson's
    - Diabetic neuropathy
    - Obesity
    - Multiple pregnancies
    - Dementia
    - Spinal cord injury
    - Stroke
- Overflow
    - Prostate enlargement (See BPH)
    - Constipation
- Functional
    - Physical disability
    - Dementia

Medications to Know

- Anticholinergics AKA antimuscarinic
    - Tolterodine, oxybutynin, solifenacin, darafenacin, trospium
    - Oxybutynin comes in a patch formulation (and oral)
        - Least selective, higher incidence on systemic anticholinergic effects
        - Cognitive impairment, constipation, urinary retention, dry eyes, dry mouth, increase fall risk
    - Other, more bladder selective agents may be more expensive
    - Make sure these drugs are actually effective, if not, try another agent or discontinue to avoid possible adverse effects
- Beta agonist (mirabegron)
    - Does have some selectivity for bladder receptors, but systemic side effects still possible
    - Can increase pulse/blood pressure
- Botox
    - Can help with spasms
    - Significant expense associated
- Topical estrogen
- Duloxetine

Urinary Tract Infections

Signs/Symptoms/Diagnosis/Complications
- Urinary frequency
- Painful or burning when urinating
- Foul, cloudy type urine (change in consistency)
- Blood tinged urine
- Pelvic or back pain (maybe more likely if kidney involvement)
- Fever, possibly less likely to spike in an elderly patient
- Cognition changes in the elderly
    - Confusion, changes in behavior
- As infection ascends into kidney, patients will generally become sicker (fever, fatigue, chills, nausea and vomiting etc.)
    - Sepsis risk increases
- Midstream catch of urine is important to avoid contamination of sample
- Routine screening via urinalysis is rarely if ever appropriate
    - 10^5 bacteria in the urine and no symptoms is ASB (Asymptomatic bacteriuria) – In general this should NOT be treated with antibiotics
    - Urinalysis (aka follow up U/A) following a course of antibiotics is also not appropriate
- UTI's most commonly caused by gram negative bacteria
    - E Coli is the most common cause (gram negative)
- If gram positive, staph saprophyticus is a common one
- Prophylaxis should be considered for patients who have recurrent UTI's
- Recurrent UTI defined as
    - > or equal to 2 infections in 6 months or > or equal to 3 in one year

Common Risk Factors
- Women
- Sexual activity
- Elderly
- Catheter
- Recent urinary surgery or anatomic changes that make infection more likely
- Immunocompromised

Medications to Know
- Sulfamethoxazole/trimethoprim

- o Beware the sulfa allergy
- o Common adverse effects; GI, rash
- o Notorious drug interaction with warfarin
- o Trimethoprim can interact with K+ elevating meds to cause hyperkalemia (i.e. ACE, ARBs, Aldosterone antagonists)
- o Drink with a glass of water
  - ▪ Crystalluria risk
- o Dose adjustments in CKD
- o Good gram negative coverage
- o Possibly some resistance depending upon the area
- Quinolones
  - o Levofloxacin/ciprofloxacin
  - o A little broader spectrum
  - o Good gram negative coverage
  - o Boxed warnings for tendon rupture etc.
  - o Drug interactions with warfarin
  - o QTC prolongation risk
  - o Dose adjustments based upon kidney function
  - o Binding interactions with cations (iron, calcium etc.)
- Nitrofurantoin
  - o Need to avoid if poor kidney function which can be a significant number of elderly patients
    - ▪ Clinicians may disagree as far as what CrCl is acceptable to use in (<30 mls/min is contraindicated for sure at this time)
  - o Educate about change in urine color (brownish/orange)
  - o Rare side effects
    - ▪ CNS changes in the elderly, especially with poor kidney function
    - ▪ Neuropathy
    - ▪ Respiratory distress
- Ceftriaxone
  - o 3rd generation cephalosporin
  - o Improved gram negative coverage over first/second generation cephalosporins
  - o Injection only
  - o Small risk of cross reaction in patients with penicillin allergy
- Cephalexin
  - o Good option if gram positive identified
  - o Not first line as far as empiric therapy
  - o GI side effects
  - o Frequent dosing is a downside

- Vaginal estrogen therapy
    - Used for prophylaxis
    - Helps maintain a normal flora to prevent infection
- Cranberry
    - Used for prophylaxis/prevention
    - Controversial as far as benefit
    - Well tolerated in most patients so often tried as a low risk option
- Other antibiotics may be used as well for treatment depending upon severity of infection and bacteria involved

Critical Guidelines/References/Resources

- Infectious Disease Society of America
- American Heart Association/American College of Cardiology
- JNC-8 Guidelines
- GOLD Guidelines
- American College of Gastroenterology
- ACIP
- FDA
- ADA
- American Geriatric Society
- American Academy of Neurology
- American College of Rheumatology
- NHLBI
- CDC
- Alzheimer's Association
- American Psychiatric Association
- DSM
- American Epilepsy Society
- American Urological Society
- WHO
- ACOG
- American Academy of Family Physicians
- AACE
- CHEST Guidelines
- American Academy of Dermatology
- KDOQI/KDIGO
- The National Kidney Foundation
- ASCO
- NCCN
- American Academy of Otolaryngologists

CPSIA information can be obtained
at www.ICGtesting.com
Printed in the USA
BVOW05s0851191216
471220BV00034B/1378/P